Perimenopause—
Preparing for the Change

Perimenopause—
Preparing for the Change
REVISED 2ND EDITION

A Guide to the Early Stages of Menopause and Beyond

Nancy Lee Teaff, M.D.
Kim Wright Wiley

THREE RIVERS PRESS
NEW YORK

Warning—Disclaimer
This book is not intended to provide medical advice and is sold with the understanding that the publisher and the author are not liable for the misconception or misuse of information provided. The author and Prima Publishing shall have neither liability nor responsibility to any person or entity with respect to any loss, damage, or injury caused or alleged to be caused directly or indirectly by the information contained in this book or the use of any products mentioned. Readers should not use any of the products discussed in this book without the advice of a medical professional.

Published in the United States by Three Rivers Press, an imprint of the Crown Publishing Group, a division of Random House, Inc., New York.
www.crownpublishing.com

THREE RIVERS PRESS and the Tugboat design are registered trademarks of Random House, Inc.

Originally published by Prima Publishing, Roseville, California, in 1999.

Products mentioned are trademarks of their respective companies.

Library of Congress Cataloging-in-Publication Data

Teaff, Nancy Lee.
    Perimenopause : preparing for the change : a guide to the early stages of menopause and beyond / Nancy Lee Teaff, Kim Wright Wiley.
    —Rev. 2nd ed
    p.   cm.
    Includes bibliographical references and index.
    1. Perimenopause—Popular works.   I. Wiley, Kim Wright.   II. Title.
RG188.T43   1999
618.1'75—dc21   99-35567
                                                                        CIP

ISBN 0-7615-1928-9
ISBN 978-0-7615-1928-7

Printed in the United States of America

10 9 8

Second Edition

To our daughters: Julia, Mary Kate, and Leigh

Contents

3   *Symptoms and Solutions*   33

4   *Hormone Replacement Therapy*   55

5 Natural Remedies for Menopausal Symptoms   83

Foreword

I am pleased to be asked to introduce the revised edition of this valuable contribution to the women's health literature. Over the past decade there has been a growing awareness of the paucity of information for women about the normal hormonal progression in midlife. In spite of an increased emphasis on finding "natural" solutions to the symptoms that arise, much of the information that is available deals with the risks and benefits of hormone therapy. Many practitioners, more oriented to disease than preventive care, are either unprepared or too busy to answer all the questions which women pose. This book helps to fill the void.

In addition to being a valuable guide for women embarking on the "menopausal transition" this book should be of help to those who have completed this life stage and need some closure for what may have been a confusing or frightening experience as well as the significant others who support and endure. The discovery that one is merely normal after all can be very beneficial.

Nancy Lee Teaff and Kim Wright Wiley have addressed the life issues of women in their 40s and 50s including the important physical and emotional changes which occur as the ovaries produce less estrogen. Subjects such as fertility potential, contraceptive needs, symptoms of declining hormone production, risks and benefits of hormone replacement therapy, and preventive measures to improve general health are addressed in an enjoyable and lucid style. In this new edition the authors also discuss alternative therapies and review the data to support their use.

This information allows the woman to take charge of her own care with confidence. Menopause is a change and there are challenges to master. These can be weathered with grace and style by the well-informed traveler who has an excellent guidebook, such as *Perimenopause—Preparing for the Change,* and a sense of humor.

Mary G. Hammond, M.D.
Reproductive Consultants, Raleigh, N.C.
past president, American Society
  for Reproductive Medicine

Preface

Kim's Story

In the five years since Nancy and I wrote the first version
of this book, there have been some major changes in my
life. My husband and I divorced after 14 years, leaving me
a part-time single parent to my thirteen-year-old daughter and 10-year-old son. Although their father and I share
custody and he is very involved in the children's lives,
there were many nights after the separation when I
prowled the house wondering "Is there going to be
enough money? Enough time to both do my job and raise
these kids? More to the point, am I enough?"

Soon after I began dating a younger man. Much
younger. (Okay, okay, fourteen years younger.) Being
with Greg challenged all my previous assumptions about
aging and age categories, and I've ricocheted through the
last few years, at times feeling like a teenager, at other

times feeling ancient. Clearly I'm having the Mother-of-All-Midlife Crises. Each morning I halfway expect to look out into my driveway and see a red Mazda Miata parked there.

Finally, and with tragic irony, in the past five years both Nancy and I have watched our mothers battle breast cancer. Now certain health issues are no longer theoretical for me; having such a scary disease hit right in your own family changes everything. Suddenly this stuff isn't just going to happen down the road someday, or happen to some woman you see on *Oprah*. Suddenly this stuff is happening here and now.

As I approached my 40s and was writing the first version of this book, I was constantly juggling. Juggling work and kids and husband and community service and personal time and searching for that mythic thing called "balance" that was supposed to let me have it all. By the time I rounded the corner into midlife, I'd had it, all right. A few of the balls were dropping and I don't think it was because I wasn't trying hard enough or was inherently clumsy. It's just that, like many American women, in my 30s I kept a pace that is impossible to sustain forever.

As you move through your 40s, it's all about reevaluating. Where I used to think "Can I do this? How can I fit it in?" I now think "Does this really matter? Can I let it go?" Certain responsibilities, such as your children, your job, and your ailing parents cannot be set aside, but during my decade-long juggling act, all the balls looked the same size to me. I couldn't separate the essential things from the non-essential, couldn't decide which balls were droppable.

The key to successfully navigating midlife is plenty of self-nurturing. I think at this point you begin to suspect that no one else can do it for you, a realization that begins as a kick in the gut and ends as a kick in the butt. It leaves you free to do the work of midlife—clearing out the stuff that doesn't fit anymore, spending time doing things you genuinely enjoy, being selective and mindful about where your energy goes. On a trip to a spa out west last year, I met a wonderful older woman who was the epitome of everything you'd want to be at seventy—a painter, hiker, world traveler, chef. As we hiked the canyons one morning, one of the younger women asked her how she stayed so amazingly vital.

"There's no secret, no one special way," she said, and we walked on in silence, because I don't think anyone had expected her to hand us a neatly-wrapped answer. But after a while she added, almost as if she were talking to herself, "But I can tell you this. When people start calling you selfish, you're on the right track." Now she wasn't a selfish person at all, no more than you or I are, but women are so accustomed to putting everyone and everything ahead of themselves that the simple question "What do I want?" can sound shallow and selfish. Ask it anyway.

Nancy's Story

What a difference four years makes! When Kim and I wrote the first edition of *Perimenopause: Preparing for the Change* we had to explain the whole concept of the process of a transition into menopause—no one had ever heard of perimenopause. Now, almost every woman's magazine has had an article on the subject. The baby boomers are reaching their 40s and 50s and are telling the world. As we predicted, perimenopause and menopause are the "Next Big Thing," as evidenced by the bookstore shelves full of how-to books on approaching this phase of a woman's life.

My own life has been busier than ever since we published the first edition of this book, especially because I believe in practicing what I preach. I've added more exercise time to my schedule, but have reduced my community commitments to spend more time with my family. (They may not agree that I'm actually spending more time at home!) I lost my mother to breast cancer this year and am having to confront my own decisions about HRT and lifestyle changes for the future. As my stage of life mirrors that of my teenage daughters, tempers sometimes flare, but overall they "grin and bear" the fact that their mother has written a book about perimenopause.

Much has changed in the past four years, but much has remained the same. HRT has been shown to be even more beneficial than earlier believed in improving the quality of life for midlife women; we now know it helps prevent Alzheimer's disease and colon cancer in addition to heart disease and osteoporosis, and no "smoking gun" has been found in the relationship between HRT and breast cancer. However, more women are seeking alternatives to HRT than ever before, so in this edition we explore alternative medicine therapies and try to give some perspective on how to incorporate them into an overall approach to wellness. We also introduce the newer medical therapies, including SERMs, to make it clear that there is an HRT regimen for everyone who needs one.

As in our first book, our agenda is to educate and inform, not to scare or intimidate women into any specific way of thinking. Women must take responsibility for their own health and not depend on the medical profession to do it for them—hence our increased emphasis on weight control, diet, and exercise. Exercise, eat right, get adequate rest, and . . . NO WHINING!

The ultimate question we should ask ourselves is "When I'm eighty, where do I want to be—in a nursing home or on a cruise ship?" I plan to tour the South Pacific myself, but what about you? Preparing for the Change starts with a little effort and education now, with the payoff of a healthy, energetic future well into your Platinum years. Let's get going!

1

Perimenopause: Preparing for the Change

This is a world of action, and not for moping and groaning in.
—Charles Dickens

We women baby boomers have had unprecedented control over our reproductive lives. Unlike our mothers and grandmothers, we've been able to decide how many children we will have, when we will have them, and—thanks to the prevalence of Lamaze and other widely taught methods and support systems—to some extent even how we will have them. At the very least, the generation of women approaching menopause today has come to expect complete access to all the facts when making their medical decisions. Often they expect almost total control.

But although we've been able to control so much about our reproductive lives, two aspects remain out of our hands: when it begins and when it ends. Menarche and menopause seem to thrust themselves upon us with a timing all their own, leaving us mumbling, "Wait, I'm not ready."

Although we can't control the when of menopause, we will, because of our sheer numbers, be able to control the how. Within the next decade, 21 million women will enter menopause, which practically guarantees that as baby boomers go through "the change" it will be a medical media event—the Next Big Thing. In 1900, fewer than 5 million women in this country were older than 50. By 2000, more than 50 million women in the United States will be over 50, making us the largest group of women to ever hit menopause at the same time.

The prototype of the menopausal woman is changing drastically. A 50-year-old American woman today is statistically likely to be working, may have young children still in the home, and, more than any previous generation, is responsible for the care of her own aging parents. The image of the granny rocking on the porch is ludicrously outdated, and the standard advice given to menopausal women 30 years ago—"Just lie down until you feel better"—simply doesn't work for a woman with a full-time job, a five-year-old child, and a mother living in her guest room. "I can't have down time," says a 48-year-old surgical nurse with three teenagers. "I can't even afford a down week."

Not only will we be going through the change in astounding numbers, but our generation will be menopausal for decades. If you menstruate from age 12 to age 49 and live to be 80 (the average life expectancy for women born in the 1950s), you'll spend half of your adult life in menopause. When you consider how much time and energy we've devoted to preparing ourselves for relatively transient sexual passages such as pregnancy, it clearly behooves us to learn as much as possible about menopause.

What Is Perimenopause?

Perimenopause means the years surrounding menopause ("peri" as in "perimeter"). Perimenopause is best defined as the transition between the time you begin to experience menopausal symptoms, usually the mid- to late 40s, and the time when your periods actually stop, the average age being 51. Some women develop symptoms in their 30s, so perimenopause can last as long as 15 years, but a more typical length is 6 years.

The term *perimenopause* has entered our vocabulary because of the increasing awareness that menopause is not an event, but a process. The ovaries begin producing less consistent levels of estrogen when a woman is in her 30s and by her mid-40s she may be experiencing symptoms of estrogen withdrawal, such as hot flashes or mood swings, even though actual menopause (cessation of menstruation) is still a decade away. Because many women define menopause as the point at which their periods stop, a woman with these early symptoms probably will not link them to hormonal changes. She's apt to dismiss her irritability or memory lapses as the result of stress, aging, or a case of "PMS from hell."

Even if she does become concerned enough to visit her doctor, she may well be told she's too young to be in menopause. Some physicians are more alert to the symptoms of perimenopause than others, but many doctors still maintain that you're either "in" menopause or you aren't —and if you're still having periods, lady, you aren't "in" anything, no matter how many hot flashes you've had. To put it mildly, not all members of the medical community are experts on this issue, so it's wise to take perimenopause into your own hands by being well-informed, alert to changes in your body, and, ultimately, willing to search for a physician who is on the same wavelength.

When Will Perimenopause Occur?

Although it would be reassuring to think you could sit down with a calculator and chart, add, and subtract all the individual factors, and then hit the total button and say "Aha, I'll enter menopause at 48," the truth is that it is extremely difficult to predict when menopause will begin for an individual woman. Certain natural variables, such as race or body type, affect when you'll go through menopause, as do lifestyle variables such as the age at which you had your first child, past illnesses or surgeries, and whether or not you smoke.

There's a common misconception that women who begin their periods earlier than average will begin menopause earlier than average, and, conversely, that women who didn't begin having periods until they were 14 or 15 will probably be well into their 50s before they experience menopause. This is a tempting theory to accept, both because it makes the onset of menopause easier to predict and because it only seems fair to assume that the first people to board the reproductive school bus in the morning would be the first ones to get off in the afternoon. Alas, the route is nowhere near as regular. Research shows no correlation between the age of menarche and the age of menopause.

Another old theory holds more water: The odds are you'll enter menopause at about the same age as your mother did. Unfortunately, because hysterectomies were so prevalent in our mothers' generation, the age in which your mother would have naturally experienced menopause is something you may never know. Numerous other factors also must be tallied—some of them logical and some seemingly random and bizarre.

You're more apt to enter menopause early if:

♦ You're thin or small-boned.

♦ You've never had children.

♦ You're Caucasian.

♦ You smoke.

- You've had a hysterectomy, tubal ligation, or three or more abortions

- You have shorter-than-average menstrual cycles, that is, fewer than 25 days apart.

Expect a later-than-average menopause if:

- You had your first child after the age of 40.

- You've had several children. In fact, research indicates that each child you bear will delay the onset of menopause by about five months.

- You've been on birth control pills for many years.

- You've had cancer of the breast or uterus, fibroids in the uterus, or diabetes.

Any factor that has affected a woman's reproductive history could potentially modify the age at which she'll go through menopause. You and your sister may have begun life with similar genetic blueprints, but if the choices each of you have made about contraception and childbearing override your inborn similarities, she may enter menopause five years later than you do.

We have heard of a male doctor, speaking before a group of women at a seminar on PMS, rather offensively claim that the women of our generation have "tinkered with their reproductive capabilities." Although we would not describe contraception, abortion, or a decision to delay childbearing as "tinkering," it is true that the track record of our older female relatives won't tell the whole story for us. For starters, we have borne fewer children and thus have had more menstrual cycles than any previous generation. And if you consider that for centuries women married shortly after puberty and remained either pregnant or nursing for most of their fertile lives, it's clear that a woman living today has had more periods than a woman living 200 years ago. Will the number of menstrual cycles a woman has in her lifetime ultimately affect when or how she enters menopause? No one knows yet, but such questions only throw more variables into the pot.

Your best approach is to be aware of the influencing factors, but not overly dependent upon them for guidance. Familiarize yourself with the harbingers of perimenopause, so that you can recognize them when they appear. The bottom line is that you don't go through menopause when the charts say you will. You go through it when you go through it.

The Life Cycle of the Ovary

Menopause may culminate in the uterus, but it begins in the ovary. Six months without periods (amenorrhea) is the most recognized clinical definition of menopause, which means that the symptom by which we diagnose menopause is actually one of the last steps in the process. The sometimes abrupt cessation of menstruation led to the euphemism "the change," as if a woman awakes one morning to find herself menopausal. But this obvious symptom was preceded by many less-noticeable pauses in ovarian function, and an overemphasis on skipped periods as the chief indicator of "the change" is one reason perimenopause is so often ignored.

The Egg Count

We've said that menopause is a process that begins before you're aware of it, but would you believe it starts before birth? In some ways, the blueprint for a woman's menopause is established when she's an embryo. By the time a female fetus reaches 20 weeks of gestation, her ovaries have a fixed number of follicles containing eggs. The number of eggs a female fetus contains drops throughout the pregnancy from a high of 2 million to the approximately 700,000 viable eggs a baby girl has at birth.

As the child grows, the eggs contained in her ovarian follicles continue to dissolve. By puberty she has approximately 400,000 left, still a staggering number, but because only one follicle of a stimulated group of follicles will mature and release an egg, the young woman can expect to experience "only" about 500 ovulations in her lifetime. The other eggs, which are not ovulated, continue to dissolve over time, even when a woman is pregnant or on the Pill.

By the time menopause approaches, the ovaries have begun to run out of the follicles that respond to the follicle-stimulating hormone (known as FSH), which prepares the follicles for ovulation. FSH causes one follicle to grow and the egg within it to mature. The layer of cells within the follicle secrete estradiol, the body's natural form of estrogen, which in turn causes the uterine lining to thicken in anticipation of receiving a fertilized egg. The stage of the menstrual cycle that precedes ovulation is the follicular phase; if there isn't a follicle healthy enough to respond to FSH, no estrogen is produced. Without estrogen, the uterine lining doesn't thicken, and there is nothing to slough off as a period.

Because FSH is such a key player in the ovulation and menstrual process, its measurement is an important indicator in how close a woman is to menopause. It's a bit confusing because a high measurement of FSH indicates menopause is approaching and a low measurement means the ovaries are still functioning. This seeming paradox is a tribute to how hard the human reproductive system strives to keep going. As menopause nears, FSH surges in a last-ditch effort to force the ovaries to release eggs—and estrogen.

A high FSH reading is considered a more accurate indicator of impending menopause than skipped periods, so if you suspect menopause is approaching you should ask your physician for an FSH test. FSH levels are checked any time from the second through the sixth day of the menstrual cycle. The actual FSH level that indicates menopause varies from one lab to another, but the general rule of thumb is that a test score higher than half of the menopausal level indicates perimenopause. In other words, if your doctor's lab defines menopause as an FSH reading of 24 and your test comes back above 12, you're moving into that borderline state of declining ovarian function known as perimenopause.

As production of estrogen and the postovulation hormone progesterone begins to taper off, the menstrual cycle will change. A previously regular woman may find herself occasionally skipping a period. Cycle length may decrease. A woman used to a 28-day cycle suddenly finds herself menstruating every 25 days.

Shorter cycles are a sign that a woman's time of ovulation has changed. As estrogen production shuts down, the number of days before cycle midpoint will decrease. As progesterone shuts down, the number of days after cycle midpoint begins to vary. If both hormones are decreased or absent, the menstrual cycle can become maddeningly unpredictable. Ovulation, which once occurred on cycle day 14 may now occur on cycle day 11—a good thing to know if you're trying to get pregnant. Or if you're not. (See Figure 1.1.)

The menstrual changes women report in perimenopause can take many forms—heavier periods, lighter periods, skipped periods, the sudden advent of PMS or cramps—but they are often the first signs that the process is underway.

Medically Induced Menopause

While we're discussing how menopause usually happens, we need to remember that not every woman enters

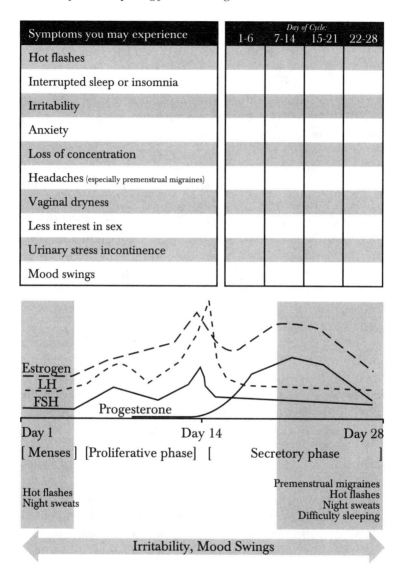

Symptoms you may experience	Day of Cycle:			
	1-6	7-14	15-21	22-28
Hot flashes				
Interrupted sleep or insomnia				
Irritability				
Anxiety				
Loss of concentration				
Headaches (especially premenstrual migraines)				
Vaginal dryness				
Less interest in sex				
Urinary stress incontinence				
Mood swings				

Estrogen
LH
FSH   Progesterone

Day 1   Day 14   Day 28
[Menses] [Proliferative phase] [Secretory phase   ]

Hot flashes
Night sweats

Premenstrual migraines
Hot flashes
Night sweats
Difficulty sleeping

Irritability, Mood Swings

Figure 1.1 Keep a record of symptoms to determine where you are in the menopausal process. The second graph shows the timing of perimenopausal symptoms related to hormonal changes during the menstrual cycle. Although irritability and mood swings may occur at any time, the other symptoms tend to center around low or falling estrogen levels.

menopause gradually. If your ovaries are removed surgically or you undergo radiation or chemotherapy treatments that are intense enough to halt ovarian function, your menopause will be immediate.

A medically induced menopause is tough for three reasons. First, your estrogen withdrawal is more abrupt than the usual winding-down process of perimenopause, so your symptoms are likely to be more dramatic as well. It's like driving a car at 60 miles per hour and suddenly slamming on the brakes. Secondly, you're already under tremendous stress due to the hysterectomy or cancer, and the unexpected addition of a whole new set of problems may seem like too much to bear. Finally, society offers virtually no support or recognition for the 31-year-old in menopause. If she's grieving over the loss of her childbearing ability or worrying about how this is going to affect her sex life, she may just be told that she's lucky to be alive at all.

It is vital for women experiencing medically induced menopause to find an empathetic doctor, one who not only can help them through the rough transition, but who is also aware of the long-term health implications of their condition. A woman going through an early menopause may be in estrogen depletion decades longer than the average woman, and because estrogen protects the heart and bones, her doctor will need to devise a program to counteract the loss.

Women in early menopause might also consider talking to a therapist or joining a support group. The standard comfort for most women in menopause is that everyone they know is going through it too. Lacking that consolation, you'll need to search harder to find women in the same boat. Many hospitals have support groups for patients recovering from cancer, and larger hospitals tend to divide the groups by age, gender, and type of illness. By talking to one another, you can share information about doctors, treatments, and coping strategies while assuaging the loneliness that often accompanies an "out of season" menopause.

How Do You Know If You're in Perimenopause?

Besides skipped periods or shorter menstrual cycles, several other symptoms indicate perimenopause. Most common are hot flashes, followed by insomnia, mood swings, loss of concentration or memory, and, finally, vaginal dryness.

We will discuss perimenopausal symptoms and suggested courses of treatment in detail in Chapter 3; the run-through here is only to help you self-diagnose the earliest stages. If you have several of the following symptoms, consider calling your doctor to schedule FSH and estradiol tests.

+ hot flashes
+ night sweats
+ interrupted sleep or insomnia
+ irritability
+ anxiety
+ loss of concentration
+ headaches (especially premenstrual migraines)
+ vaginal dryness
+ less interest in sex
+ urinary stress incontinence
+ mood swings

Obviously, many of these symptoms are interconnected. If you have such severe night sweats that you develop insomnia, your concentration will suffer and you'll be too tired for sex. From there the dominoes just keep falling, and what begins as a physical problem can escalate into a psychological one. The mood swings of perimenopause may make you feel like you're back in seventh grade, and indeed the hormonal changes of perimenopause are more like puberty than you might guess.

Reverse Puberty

In puberty, early estrogen production leads to breast development and the growth of the endometrium (uterine lining), which will ultimately shed itself and become the girl's first menstrual cycle. During the first year or two of menarche, a girl's cycles are often irregular and usually not ovulatory. Estrogen production is also erratic, and these fluctuating hormonal levels, coupled with the daily traumas of adolescent life, lead to the wild mood swings that are so much a part of being a pubescent girl.

In menopause the exact reverse happens, but with similar results. The ovaries are gearing down instead of gearing up, but the dueling hormonal levels can bring on the same mood swings a woman experienced 40 years earlier—and the same helpless feeling that makes a woman wonder, "What's happening to me?"

The key is that a consistent hormonal cycle enables a woman to predict her ups and downs. She may have PMS, but at least she knows when to expect it and can recognize it for what it is. But when the hormonal change disrupts the cycle's regularity and hormone levels rise and fall in an unpredictable pattern throughout this new non-cycle, the woman may begin to suffer bouts of irritability and depression.

Diagnostic Tests for Perimenopause

The two most important diagnostic tests for perimenopause are the FSH test and a test to check your estradiol level.

Is This PMS or Perimenopause?

Many of the symptoms of perimenopause are also symptoms of PMS, so it's easy to automatically dismiss your complaints as PMS, especially if you're still having regular periods. But you should suspect perimenopause if:

1. You never had PMS, but you suddenly start.
2. You always had PMS, but now a new symptom has kicked in, such as night sweats or headaches.
3. The symptoms don't disappear when your period starts.

PMS has cyclic, somewhat predictable patterns of symptoms, while perimenopausal symptoms are less consistent. You may feel irritable and suffer insomnia for several months and then have the problems suddenly abate, only to return six months later. Chart your mood swings in relation to your menstrual cycles. If no pattern emerges and what you seem to be having is month-long PMS, it may actually be perimenopause.

A changing menstrual pattern or hot flashes indicate that your estrogen production is slowing and an FSH test should be done. As mentioned earlier, the test is relatively simple: Blood is drawn at some time during the first two to six days of your menstrual cycle (or any time if you're not having periods) for two successive months. If your FSH levels exceed what your lab defines as menopausal levels on both occasions, the ovary is shutting down, and you're approaching menopause. As mentioned earlier, a reading of more than half of what your lab defines as the menopausal level is significant enough to suggest that you're perimenopausal. Menopause will likely occur within the next five years.

Don't be frustrated if you end up with a borderline diagnosis. Not all gynecologists even recognize FSH tests as reliable indicators, and among those who do there is a marked difference of opinion about exactly what level constitutes menopause. Furthermore, on any given cycle your FSH might be in normal ranges and on the next it could approach the menopausal range. Symptoms, especially menstrual irregularity, are the real key to diagnosing perimenopause, but the FSH test can be helpful in indicating where you are on the continuum, or, in some cases, confirming what you already suspect.

Your estrogen level affects how you feel, making the estradiol test another vital piece in the perimenopausal puzzle. (Remember that estradiol is the primary type of estrogen that the ovaries produce.) For this test, blood is drawn on day two, three, or four of the menstrual cycle to see if it's within normal ranges. Strangely enough, an inappropriately high level of estrogen also indicates the erratic ovarian function typical of perimenopause. Any deviation from the normal pattern is noteworthy.

An estradiol check alone suffices for many women, although your physician may opt for a total ovarian hormonal profile. Your testosterone level can be checked any time, and a low reading is often behind a loss of libido. If you're trying to conceive or having severe problems with menstrual irregularity, your progesterone level should be checked after ovulation is thought to have occurred, usually around days 20 to 22 of your menstrual cycle.

An Overall Health Evaluation

Other tests your doctor may suggest are only indirectly related to menopause. This is the time of life when you should begin having routine mammograms and cholesterol checks, if you aren't already. If you have a family history of cancer, especially breast, ovarian, or colon cancer, you may need to have more frequent screenings than the average woman.

One of the biggest health challenges faced by older women is osteoporosis, and your risk can be determined based on a dual energy X-ray absorptiometry (DEXA) exam, which measures your current bone mineral content. Much as an early mammogram establishes a baseline against which further screening tests are measured, an early DEXA will help your physician ascertain whether you're losing, maintaining, or building bone mass in years to come. Perimenopause is an excellent time to do such an overall health evaluation (see Figure 1.2). Your body is telling you that it's changing, and you may want to reassess how you're living in regard to nutrition, exercise, and stress. The point of this advice is not to make you feel fragile, or to suggest that you run to your doctor with the first faint symptom, but rather to encourage you to take a proactive stance toward the next 40 years of your life. And if your physician tells you that you're "too young" to be worrying about such things, step one should be to look for a new physician.

Your Medical History

Your doctor should begin by asking if you have a personal or family history of:

+ heart disease
+ breast disease
+ liver disease
+ cancer (especially if you or a close female relative has had cancer of the breast, uterus, ovary, or cervix)
+ osteoporosis
+ diabetes

Test	30–39 years	40–49 years	50–59 years
1. complete examination	every 4 years	every 4 years	every 4 years
2. blood pressure	every other year	every other year	every other year
3. breast examination	every other year	every year	every year
4. Pap smear	every other year	every other year	every other year
5. pelvic examination	every other year	every year	every year
6. mammogram	age 36	every other year	every year
7. cholesterol check	every 5 years	every 5 years	every 5 years
8. stool examination	every other year	every other year	every year
9. sigmoidoscopy	—	—	every 4 years
10. dental cleaning	twice a year	twice a year	twice a year
11. eye examination	—	—	every 3 years

Figure 1.2 Routine Healthcare Checklist

Do you have any drug allergies? What medications, vitamin supplements, or herbal supplements are you currently taking?

What about your gynecological history? Take the time to discuss your:

- menstrual patterns
- pregnancy history
- sexual history
- gynecologic operations
- current symptoms of perimenopause, if any (see Figure 1.1)

Your doctor should also discuss your current health:

- Do you smoke?
- Do you exercise on a regular basis?
- Do you watch your diet, especially in terms of getting adequate fiber and calcium?
- Are you overweight?

A thorough doctor will also take the time to utilize the most important instrument in modern medicine: the chair. You should schedule a conference time both to discuss test results and to bring up symptoms or concerns that don't fit into a previously analyzed category—a loss of energy, perhaps, or any personal problems that affect your stress level or overall health. Don't attempt to discuss perimenopause with your doctor during a routine Pap smear. This is not an "Oh, by the way" condition, and unless you schedule adequate time for a conference, you'll feel you got a rush job, which isn't fair to either you or your physician.

It's vital to assess your personal risk for the "big three:" heart disease, osteoporosis, and breast cancer. Use the lists in Chapter 6 to assess yourself. If you have several listed factors predisposing you toward a certain illness, this may warrant more frequent screenings than those routinely recommended and more aggressive preventive care.

Obviously, not every factor carries equal weight—a family history of breast cancer under the age of 50 is much more a cause for concern than merely being Caucasian. But the lists are helpful in making you aware of where you are potentially at risk.

Why Should You Care?

Why should we become so hypersensitive about the approach of menopause? A quick scan of the symptoms may convince you that you suffer all of them—and have, frankly, since birth. You may feel so worn down from the sheer weight of the issues that you're tempted to think, "I'll just get through menopause, whenever it comes. Everybody does, including my own mother, who to my knowledge never even uttered the word aloud."

The main reason to arm yourself with knowledge now is so you can take a proactive stance. As we've seen, by the time symptoms become apparent, changes have been going on for months or years beneath the surface. And by the time symptoms become genuinely disruptive, you will have missed several opportunities to intervene.

From 15 to 20 percent of women going through menopause report symptoms severe enough to disrupt their ability to function at home or at work, while 65 to 80 percent report noticeable symptoms beyond skipped periods. Granted, these complaints are rarely crippling, but why suffer from them any more than you have to? Going to your doctor only when your symptoms become unbearable is simply not good preventive medicine and certainly not a smart choice for a woman who needs to function at peak capacity every day of the month.

If we've learned anything from the women we interviewed for this book, it's that the women who most successfully handle perimenopause meet the condition head-on, persisting even in the face of bewildering symptoms and a sometimes indifferent medical community. Consider the fact that you'll likely be menopausal for decades and ask yourself if you really want to "tough it out" for 40 years. If you enter perimenopause with no information at all, you'll undoubtedly survive, but how good are you going to feel? For women of our generation, how well we prepare for menopause may be the ultimate quality-of-life issue.

2

❧

Fertility and Infertility

You can't always get what you want . . . but you just might find you get what you need.

—*You Can't Always Get What You Want*
by the Rolling Stones

Call it Murphy's Law of Perimenopause: The women who want to get pregnant can't, and those who don't want to get pregnant do. The cruel irony is that the number of forty-something women thronging to the infertility clinics is exceeded only by the number of forty-something women thronging to the abortion clinics.

Surprisingly, women in their 40s have the second highest rate of unplanned pregnancies of any age group. Only teenage girls goof more often than we do—and only teenage girls have more abortions.

Why do mature women get pregnant so often by mistake? It's obviously not because they're carried away on a tide of passion in the backseat of a car, but more likely because they didn't realize they were still fertile. Women commonly misinterpret skipped periods as the absence of ovulation, or fail to realize that during perimenopause a woman can produce a nonviable egg in one cycle and a viable egg in the next, essentially rotating between fertility and infertility.

To be absolutely safe, most doctors recommend maintaining contraception for a full year after your last menstrual cycle. This may sound like paranoia, but it's actually self-protective. The challenges of menopause are intense enough without adding a surprise pregnancy to the mix.

How to Tell If You're Ovulating

As we discussed in Chapter 1, the reproductive cycle is not a roulette wheel that is stopped in midspin by the hand of fate. Egg production winds down slowly.

Although men produce sperm throughout their lives, a woman is born with all the eggs she'll ever have. The eggs die off at a rate of about 1,000 per month, but because we begin life with as many as 700,000 eggs, the perimenopausal woman still has about 10,000 eggs left, technically more than enough. As we near menopause, however, the follicle may fail to release an egg each month. Even if it is released, the egg itself is now more than 40 years old and may no longer be viable. (The egg is living, but by viable we mean capable of being fertilized and attaching itself to the uterine wall.) Eight out of every 10 eggs a woman over the age of 40 ovulates are genetically abnormal and unlikely to be fertilized, which is bad news for the perimenopausal woman who is trying to conceive, because every missed cycle is a missed opportunity.

But the equally bad news if you're trying *not* to get pregnant is that this same theoretical woman is producing viable eggs during some months of the year. Natural menopause has occurred in only 11 percent of women aged 45 to 49, so unless she's had surgical intervention, a woman in her late 40s should assume that she is still potentially fertile.

If you have doubts about whether you're still fertile, an FSH test will give you more to go on. An FSH reading that falls in the range your doctor considers menopausal indicates that you have virtually no chance of conceiving. Any FSH reading of greater than one-half the number your doctor considers to be indicative of menopause means your chances of conceiving have dropped to around 5 percent. If you're sure you don't want a pregnancy and are unwilling to take a 1-in-20 chance of conceiving, continue to use contraception.

How to Get Pregnant

Over the last 20 years, the number of women over 35 who are giving birth for the first time has increased dramatically. The tendency to marry later and delay childbearing has resulted in many more 35- to 44-year-old women who are trying to either start a family or expand their family as perimenopause approaches.

New Passages author Gail Sheehy refers to women in their 40s who are attempting pregnancy for the first time as "the great postponers," with the "fantasy of fertility forever." It sounds a bit pejorative, perhaps, but it's a fair characterization of the way some women think. The myth that it's a snap to conceive in midlife is fueled by the pictures of smiling forty-something actresses cuddling their newborns on the cover of women's magazines, but the reality is that these high-profile women probably had some high-tech help.

Clinically, infertility is defined as the inability to conceive within one year. The standard advice is if you've gone a year with unprotected sex and still aren't pregnant, there's a 90 percent chance that something is wrong and you need medical attention.

A woman over 35, however, can't afford to wait a full year before seeking help. There are numerous infertility treatments in use today, but many of them take time. As soon as she decides she wants a baby, a woman over 35 should begin using ovulation predictor kits or basal body temperature (BBT) charting, and if six months of intercourse scheduled at the time of ovulation don't result in pregnancy, she should schedule a consultation.

The time factor plays out as follows: The risk of infertility rises from 6 percent for women between ages 20 and 24 to 64 percent for women between 40 and 44. Put another way, within 10 months of trying, 80 percent of women under 34 will get pregnant on their own. (Well, they will need a man or, at least, sperm.) But only 4 percent of women over 40 conceive within 10 months without any sort of medical intervention.

This doesn't mean that if you're in your 40s you aren't still fertile, particularly if you've already given birth. For some reason, having babies before the age of 40 improves the odds of having a baby after 40. However, your chances of conceiving are greater at 40 than 42, and greater at 42 than 44. If a friend with no kids becomes pregnant at 43, the chances are high that she's using a donor egg. (But it's not polite to ask!)

It's your rate of fecundity—the chance of conception during a single menstrual cycle—that falls so sharply in your 40s. There are several reasons:

1. First and foremost, the quality and the number of your eggs has diminished. Sorry to keep harping, but women seem determined to downplay the severity of this problem.

2. Couples in their 40s tend to have sex less frequently than couples in their 20s. You gotta play to win.

3. Inadequate progesterone production may result in a deficient preparation of the endometrium. If the uterine lining isn't ready, the fertilized egg can't implant and no pregnancy results. This condition is sometimes referred to as luteal phase deficiency.

4. Endometriosis is common among women in their 40s. Normally, the endometrium either receives the fertilized egg and provides nourishment for an embryo, or, if no fertilization has taken place, it is shed during the period. In endometriosis, the uter-

ine lining leaks out through the fallopian tubes and into the pelvic cavity. It can then adhere to the ovaries and to the outside of the uterus, not only preventing conception but also causing extreme discomfort.

5. Tubal infertility (damaged fallopian tubes) is another potential problem. If the problem is minimal, such as slight scarring, laparoscopic surgery can be performed on an outpatient basis. If the damage is more severe, in vitro fertilization (IVF) becomes the treatment of choice, because it bypasses the fallopian tubes altogether.

A reduction in fecundity doesn't occur only in women. Only one-third of males over the age of 40 manage to impregnate their partner within six months. Although many of the causes of male infertility, such as undescended testicles or diseases such as mumps, are present from childhood, environmental factors can also be responsible: A man who previously fathered a child may find himself entering middle age with a reduced sperm count.

An Infertility Consultation: What to Expect

A typical fertility workup begins with both partners giving their complete medical—and sexual—histories. Standard tests include a semen analysis for the man, a hormonal evaluation for the woman, and a postcoital test to study the interaction between the man's sperm and the woman's cervical mucus. A hysterosalpingogram (HSG) sounds dreadful but is actually a relatively simple X-ray procedure during which dye is injected into the uterus to see whether it flows through the fallopian tubes, indicating whether or not they are blocked.

If the woman is over 35, the physician may also schedule a laparoscopy as part of the initial workup. Ordinarily a laparoscopy, which allows direct observation of the ovaries and fallopian tubes through a small incision made below the navel, is delayed until an HSG indicates an abnormality. But because the HSG cannot detect all problems and even the slightest degree of endometriosis or scar tissue can interfere with an already tenuous fertility, a physician may schedule a laparoscopy earlier for an older woman.

On the other hand, if the woman's HSG is normal and she has no symptoms of endometriosis, the doctor could suggest she go directly to IVF, which is less invasive than laparoscopy and would directly address the objective of getting pregnant. With IVF success rates approaching 50 percent per cycle for women aged 35 to 39, fertility specialists are recommending this option more often and skipping the laparoscopy. The choice should be individualized for each patient, but the reality is that you don't always have to know the cause of the infertility to successfully treat it.

Finally, your doctor may order a clomiphene citrate challenge test (CCCT). *Ovarian reserve* is a term referring to the reproductive potential of a woman based on the number and quality of eggs remaining in her ovaries, and it can give you an estimate of how many "baby-grade" eggs you have left. An FSH level is checked on cycle day 3, and the patient takes clomiphene citrate (brand names: Clomid, Serophene) on cycle days 5 through 9. Another FSH is taken on cycle day 10. An abnormally elevated value on either day indicates a decreased ovarian reserve.

Ninety-five percent of infertility patients who have an abnormal CCCT will be unable to deliver a baby even with ovulation induction or IVF. They may become pregnant, but they are extremely likely to miscarry. Even with a normal CCCT, women over 40 have a lower conception rate than 35-year-old women, but a normal CCCT indicates that an older woman is a reasonable candidate for high-tech infertility treatments.

Infertility Treatments

The method of treatment, of course, depends on the reason for the infertility. If a total absence of sperm is the problem, donor insemination will be advised; the success rate for women over 35 using donor sperm is high, with 54 percent conceiving over a span of 12 cycles. If your partner has a very low sperm count, you may want to consider a procedure called intracytoplasmic sperm injection (ICSI), an extension of IVF where your partner's sperm is placed directly inside the egg to accomplish fertilization. ICSI has success rates equal to those of standard IVF treatments for any given age group.

If blocked fallopian tubes or endometriosis are the root of the problem, these conditions can often be corrected through laparoscopic surgery or IVF.

Even if her CCCT is normal, a woman over age 40 should prepare herself for intensive fertility treatment. Injectable fertility drugs (brand names: Gonal f, Follistim, Repronex, Pergonal, Humegon) force the ovary to produce as many eggs as possible in a cycle. These drugs are often coupled with intrauterine insemination (IUI), a treatment that injects the man's washed sperm into the woman's uterus. This technique is a pure numbers game: You're trying to get the most eggs the woman is capable of producing in contact with the greatest number of sperm the man can offer, and do this as close to the time of ovulation as possible.

As age becomes a factor, a treatment is evaluated not only in terms of how well it works, but also how quickly it works. Given the catch-22 of perimenopausal fertility—it takes more time to get pregnant and you have less time—in vitro fertilization and similar procedures are often recommended because they have the highest per cycle likelihood of producing a pregnancy.

If your CCCT is abnormal, the chances of success using your own eggs is remote. Now is the time to reconsider exactly why you want a child: Are you seeking to reproduce yourself genetically? Do you want the experiences of pregnancy and birth? Or do you simply long to be a parent and the method by which you receive the child is incidental? If your primary objective is parenthood and not necessarily pregnancy, you can—and should—consider a wider range of options, such as adoption. But if you strongly desire the birth experience, then it's literally back to the lab for you.

High-Tech Pregnancies

An increasingly common form of assisted pregnancy is IVF or in vitro fertilization, popularly known as a "test-tube baby." Either the woman's own egg or a donor's egg is removed from a ripe follicle and fertilized by a sperm cell outside the body. The fertilized egg is allowed to grow and divide for several days before it is inserted into the woman's uterus.

When a woman decides she wants to try IVF, her first decision is whether to use her own eggs. Understandably, most women prefer giving their own eggs a try before using those of a donor, but you should consider this only if your CCCT is normal. The IVF success rate is less than 5 percent per cycle when a woman over the age of 40 with an abnormal CCCT uses her own eggs. In contrast, the success rate is about 50 percent per cycle (or higher) using donor eggs. Given the expense and invasiveness of the treatments, many physicians encourage women with an abnormal CCCT to use donor eggs from the start.

Depending upon the condition of your eggs and your partner's sperm, there are four ways to make a high-tech baby:

1. *Your egg and your partner's sperm.*
   If you have viable eggs and your partner has viable sperm, the resulting baby will be a genetic mix of

the two of you, albeit mixed in a slightly unusual container.

2. *Your eggs and a donor's sperm.*
   For women with viable eggs who either have no partner or a partner with no viable sperm, donor sperm can be used. A variation on artificial insemination, IVF is an option for the woman who is pushing either the age or the estrogen limit but still has some healthy eggs left, or one whose fallopian tubes are damaged.

3. *Donor eggs and your partner's sperm.*
   If your ovary is faltering, but your partner has viable sperm, you can use a donor egg. The uterus soldiers on for several years after the ovary has retired, so pregnancy is possible even for a woman who is menopausal.

4. *Donor eggs and donor sperm.*
   Even if your eggs and your partner's sperm are both nonviable, you can still have the pregnancy and birth experience with conception via IVF.

If you are exhibiting signs of perimenopause but want to have a child, you probably cannot simply let nature take its course. We often speak of people as being simply fertile or infertile, but there is a third category between the two, "subfertile," and many perimenopausal women fall into it. If you wait too long to seek medical help you may end up needing more invasive and complex treatment than you would if you'd gone in earlier. The payoff in reacting quickly to signs of subfertility is that you have more options, more time, and thus a greater chance of having a baby.

Note: All this talk about "partners" and "husbands" is a matter of linguistic convenience, and is not meant to disparage a single woman's attempts to achieve motherhood. The obvious truth is that you don't need a husband or even a male partner in order to get pregnant. You need only sperm, and, luckily, they're not hard to obtain.

The basic question for a single woman is the same as for her married counterpart: Are your eggs viable? If they are, you can seek pregnancy through artificial insemination. If not, you'll require both donor sperm and eggs and will need to investigate IVF.

How to Stay Pregnant

Once the fertilized egg attaches to the uterine wall, the perimenopausal mother faces another hurdle. The risk of spontaneous abortion, or miscarriage, increases significantly as a woman ages. A 30-year-old woman has a 10 percent chance of miscarriage, rising to a 33 percent risk for women aged 40 to 44; a woman over the age of 45 is more likely to miscarry than to bring a pregnancy to term. FSH can be a barometer of how apt you are to miscarry: A high FSH level at any age portends a greater likelihood of miscarriage.

Furthermore, babies born to older mothers bear a well-publicized risk of chromosomal abnormalities. Amniocentesis and chronic villus sampling (CVS) are recommended for women who will be 35 or older at the time of birth. CVS diagnoses a range of genetic abnormalities, and is done around the tenth to twelfth week of pregnancy. Amniocentesis involves withdrawal of fluid from the amniotic sac and is performed around the sixteenth week. If you're concerned about birth defects, ask your physician for a referral to a genetic counselor, who can discuss your options for prenatal diagnosis.

If a woman over 40 begins pregnancy without a high-risk factor working against her, has the early screening tests, and does not miscarry, she will likely deliver a healthy baby. The horror stories about older mothers are often linked to preexisting medical conditions such as diabetes, hypertension, and obesity, or a family history of genetic abnormalities. A healthy 40-year-old with good prenatal care can expect a positive outcome.

How Not to Get Pregnant

Of course, if you don't want to have a baby, all of the statistics in the previous sections can be inverted. A woman in her late 30s who is using no contraception has a 30 to 50 percent chance of conceiving—so this is no time to get sloppy about birth control. The estrogen in hormone replacement therapy (HRT) may actually increase ovarian function, and consequently increase the chances of conception.

Sterilization of one member of the couple is the most common way to prevent unwanted pregnancy in the United States; about half of married couples choose this method. In terms of reversible contraception, oral contraceptives (OCs) are the most popular, with 20 percent of women 18 to 44 using the Pill.

Using oral contraceptives has an added advantage because the Pill contains sufficient quantities of estrogen and progesterone to help control hot flashes and irregular periods, two of the most common complaints of perimenopause. Oral contraceptives in effect serve as low-dosage hormone replacement therapy, helping women maintain bone density and regular menstrual cycles, as well as protecting against pregnancy. A growing number of women opt to take the Pill throughout their 40s and then switch directly to HRT when they become menopausal.

Unless a woman smokes or has another high-risk factor, such as blood clots or previous cardiovascular disease, the benefits of remaining on oral contraceptives outweigh the risks. The Pill is safer than pregnancy, especially for women in their 40s, and women approaching perimenopause can often get away with the very lowest dosage because their ovarian function is already lessened and thus easier to control. Long-term OC use also reduces your risk of ovarian cancer, which is particularly important for women who have never had children, because ordinarily they would be at higher risk for the disease.

The Pill is followed in frequency of use by condoms, the rhythm method, withdrawal, diaphragms, IUDs, and spermicides. Other methods now available include Depo-Provera injections, the Norplant implant, and the female condom. It may surprise you to note how the clumsy attempts at contraception of the teenage years—withdrawal and the rhythm method—reassert themselves among couples in their 40s. Obviously, withdrawal and attempting to have intercourse during the "safe times" have always been risky, and become only more so when the woman is having irregular menstrual cycles. The high failure rate of these methods is reflected in the abortion statistics for women in our age group.

If you have multiple partners or your partner has multiple partners, condoms are a must, as they reduce your exposure to sexually transmitted diseases, including AIDS. The female condom is especially effective, because more of the vulva and the base of the penis are protected, thus lessening the chance of pregnancy and of transmitting herpes or genital warts. It's noteworthy that women who use diaphragms have one-third the risk of cervical cancer of women who use no such protection, possibly due to the antiviral action of the spermicide used with the diaphragm.

Remember, just because you're not ovulating regularly, don't assume that you're not ovulating at all. If there is any doubt that you are not fully menopausal, continue to use contraception.

3

Symptoms and Solutions

A problem well-defined is half-solved.

—John Dewey

There's an old cartoon that shows a husband returning home from work to find his house in shambles. Garbage is strewn all over the floor, laundry is hanging from the lamps and chairs, and the children are chasing each other around the house with flaming arrows. His wife looks up from the couch and says, "You know how you're always asking me what I do all day? Well, today I didn't do it."

Estrogen is like the housewife in the cartoon: We don't appreciate all the things it does until it stops doing them. This hormone contributes a great deal behind the scenes to maintain health, youth, and vitality; once it departs from the system, myriad symptoms can occur, ranging from the merely irritating to the severely incapacitating.

When they first begin to appear, perimenopausal symptoms may seem to be unrelated to each other, and women often treat each problem individually, not seeing the connection until years later. Skipped periods and hot flashes are almost automatically attributed to menopause, but if your first symptom happens to be insomnia or a loss of concentration, you may spend many hours in a therapist's office before it becomes apparent that the problem is primarily hormonal. And if your third and fourth symptoms are itchy skin and urinary incontinence, not only are you unlikely to link them to menopause, you're also unlikely to see their connection to the insomnia or concentration loss. A woman may say, "I'm falling apart," without recognizing that there is really only one condition, perimenopause, that is manifesting itself in many ways.

Perhaps it will help to think of perimenopause as producing a constellation of symptoms. There is a pattern, but the pattern is often evident only when you stand back and try to see it as a whole. As long as you focus on each individual star—each individual symptom—you'll miss the bigger picture (see Figure 3.1).

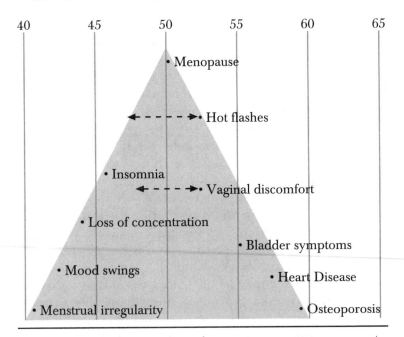

Figure 3.1 Sample timeline of symptoms in perimenopause/postmenopause.

How Bad Will the Symptoms Be?

Most women go through menopause with only minor difficulty, but about 20 to 30 percent experience symptoms that they describe as being severe enough to affect their function at home or work. There's no sure way to predict whether you'll be among those who have a rough time, although there is evidence to suggest that thin women have more pronounced symptoms than overweight women. This is due to the fact that fat cells are capable of manufacturing a type of weak estrogen called estrone, which can curb minor symptoms.

Also, as discussed in Chapter 1, the more abrupt your transition to menopause, the more dramatic your symptoms. In addition, women with a history of PMS or other menstrual difficulties report more problems with menopause than average.

HRT: The Umbrella Treatment

A majority of the symptoms we will describe in this chapter respond favorably to hormone replacement therapy (HRT). If your symptoms are bad enough to truly get you down, you should investigate the possibility of HRT, even if you're still menstruating. Hormone replacement therapy is a complex and somewhat controversial issue and will be discussed in more detail in Chapter 4.

For now it is enough to mention that HRT is the oft-prescribed umbrella treatment for women who experience multiple symptoms, simply because putting estrogen and progesterone back into the system eliminates many complaints in one fell swoop. HRT releases both the doctor and the patient from the arduous task of trying to sort out the causes of individual symptoms. A quick glance at the list of symptoms shows how interrelated many of them are—who can say if she's depressed from a lack of sleep or if she has insomnia because she's depressed? Life's problems seldom happen in a linear fashion, and because women are subject to such a wide variety of pressures, it can be downright impossible to say just which symptom came first.

But the interrelationship of the symptoms can also work in your favor, for by solving one problem you often indirectly solve others. Anything that reduces stress reduces the symptoms of perimenopause. Relaxation techniques such as massage, biofeedback, yoga, meditation or prayer, a regular sleep schedule, an exercise program, and therapy or a support group can have a great impact on how you handle perimenopause. Relaxation techniques are proactive medicine in its most potent form: You may not be able to avoid experiencing a single hot flash, but you can stop the domino effect that occurs when one symptom, unchecked, sets off another and then another.

Most women who have extreme difficulty in perimenopause have multiple symptoms, but a woman experiencing only one symptom probably won't need the entire battery of HRT to combat it. For example, if insomnia is the only thing really getting to you, try the simple suggestions in the solution section for that symptom before embarking on a treatment designed to cure a batch of ills you don't have.

Symptoms of Perimenopause

Hot Flashes

The problem: You're sitting at your desk in the afternoon when you suddenly feel warm. You remove your jacket and loosen your collar, but within minutes a red flush has risen from your chest and spread across your torso and up your neck to your scalp. You begin sweating and when you mop your brow with a tissue, you realize your makeup is coming off. After a couple of uncomfortable minutes, and a few pointed glances from the man at the desk beside you, the hot flash abates. But your blouse is soaked with perspiration, and almost immediately you begin to feel chilled.

Up to 25 percent of perimenopausal women and a whopping 50 to 85 percent of menopausal women experience hot flashes. Sometimes called a hot flush, because you do redden or blush as a result of the dilation of the blood vessels, a hot flash is a sensation of heat that begins in the face, head, or chest. Some women have a specific focal point such as an earlobe or the skin between their breasts; when they feel the first tingles there, they know a hot flash is approaching. From the initial site, the hot flash can spread over the entire body in a matter of seconds. The degree of sensation varies from mild discomfort to a feeling so intense that women have to fight the urge to pull off clothing.

Hot flashes typically last three minutes, but can range in duration from a few seconds to an entire hour. Most menopausal women experience them for only about a year; they are, in fact, one of the more transitory complaints of menopause, and one many women decide to grin and bear. But in 25 percent of women they persist for five years—too long to suffer without help.

The precise physical origin of a hot flash is not understood, but it appears to be linked to estrogen withdrawal. Among its many other functions, estrogen affects the hypothalamus, the hormone- and heat-regulating center in the brain. As menopause approaches, this internal thermostat gets out of whack, causing a sudden inappropriate activation of the body's heat-release mechanisms.

Studies show that a woman's temperature rises just slightly before a hot flash, although you may feel it's rising dramatically. One woman described it as the "exploding thermometer effect" of a cartoon. Blood vessels dilate in an attempt to cool the body, causing the familiar flush, and your body begins to sweat in an effort to lower its temperature. Once the flash passes, your pores are open and your skin is damp, setting you up for the chill that frequently follows.

Why are some women affected much more intensely than others? The answer appears to lie in how much their estrogen level varies in the course of a day. If a woman has a small, steady amount of estrogen in her system, her body adapts, but if the levels are continuously rising and falling, the body is forced to adjust repeatedly, and hot flashes become more pronounced.

The solution: Estrogen replacement is the foundation of hot-flash therapy, dating back to nineteenth century when a sheep's ovary sandwich was a prescribed remedy. This is probably where the tradition of "grin and bear it" originated.

Estrogen is now usually administered in either pill or skin-patch form, and its effect on hot flashes is swift. For women who are not good candidates for HRT, the hypertension medicine clonidine (brand name: Catapres) has proven to reduce hot flashes, as have anti-prostaglandins such as Naproxen. Soy proteins and progestins such as norethindrone have also been shown to help.

If your hot flashes are relatively mild or you'd like to avoid drug therapy, biofeedback has helped some women cope. European studies have shown that women who engage in regular aerobic exercise report only half as many hot flashes as sedentary women.

Two things that don't work: Vitamin E and dong quai were once highly touted as helpful, but in double-blind studies have proven no more effective than a placebo.

Night Sweats and Insomnia

The problem: You awake at 3:15 A.M. in the midst of a hot flash. By the time it passes, your gown and sheets are soaked. You get up, shower, change your gown, and put towels over the damp sheets in order not to disturb your husband. But after all this activity, you can't get back to sleep. At 5:21 A.M. you're still awake, and because you have to leave for work in two hours, you go ahead and get up, knowing you'll drag through the day.

Sweating often follows hot flashes. An episode that occurs at night, called a night sweat, produces an exaggerated feeling of heat, partly because our sleeping bodies beneath blankets are warmer at night and partly because if we're asleep we miss the warning tingles of an approaching flash and are unable to drink water, unbutton our collars, or do anything to diminish the impact.

These disturbances can wake you from a sound sleep, and if they happen regularly enough, the result is chronic sleep deprivation, similar to what you experience when a newborn joins the family. Achieving only shallow sleep for a couple of hours at a time is a condition known as low sleep effectiveness. Because older people are at risk for insomnia anyway, a woman plagued with night sweats faces a double whammy: It's harder for her to get to sleep and then harder for her to stay asleep. Untreated, sleep deprivation can lead to depression.

The solution: HRT helps because it both reduces the frequency and intensity of hot flashes and improves the general quality of sleep. Regular exercise can effectively battle insomnia, but don't work out within two hours of going to bed or your revved-up metabolism won't allow you to rest. It's also important to follow a routine that encourages sleep by maintaining a consistent bedtime and engaging in whatever sort of soothing ritual—a warm bath, hot milk, gentle music, or reading—works to make you drowsy.

Insomnia is also obviously linked to stress, so stress-reduction techniques—yoga, meditation, prayer, or a progressive relaxation tape—can also help you get to sleep.

Caffeine and alcohol affect people more as they get older, so even if you could have three glasses of wine and then sleep through the night 10 years ago, don't assume that your current wakefulness isn't caused by the alcohol. Smoking and some antihistamines have also proven to disrupt the sleep cycle, even in people who did not report sleep problems when they were younger. Depression is also a major cause of sleep disturbance, and if a woman doesn't respond well to HRT, she might also want to talk to her doctor about antidepressant medication.

If your insomnia does not respond to these common-sense methods, or if HRT stops the night sweats but you're still having trouble getting to sleep, you may need to visit a sleep disorder clinic or try biofeedback. For information on the center nearest you, contact the Association of Applied Biofeedback, listed in the Sources section at the end of this book.

Poor Memory and Loss of Concentration

The problem: You notice you're having trouble remembering simple things, that you have to make a list before going to the supermarket even if you need only three items. Your reaction time seems delayed and you often feel vaguely unfocused.

For a working woman or a mother who still has young children who depend upon her alertness, memory loss can be among the most upsetting symptoms of perimenopause. Short-term memory is more often affected than long term. You may look up an address and forget it before you can write it down, or go absolutely blank on the name of your child's fifth-grade teacher. One menopause support group tells a funny story of how they intended for three months to ask their visiting speakers to address the issue of memory loss—but all kept forgetting what it was they were worried about. Finally they made a banner that read, "Remember that we've lost our memory," and taped it to the meeting room wall.

One of the reasons memory loss is so scary for the menopausal woman is that she may think, "I'm cracking up," or, "I'm getting Alzheimer's." *Alzheimer's disease,* which is incorrectly used as an umbrella term for any aging-related memory loss, is a specific and debilitating illness that has nothing to do with perimenopausal loss of concentration. Alzheimer's disease is not forgetting where your keys are, it's forgetting what a key is and that you use it to lock the door.

Even your doctor may not connect your forgetfulness to estrogen loss, but may rather fuel your fears by attributing the problem to stress or aging. If you're experiencing night sweats and insomnia as well, your troubles are clearly compounded, because it's hard to stay alert if you've had only four hours of sleep the night before. Once again, the more abrupt the estrogen withdrawal, the more upsetting the symptoms, and women recovering from hysterectomies or chemotherapy often report an alarming degree of forgetfulness, which they generally fail to connect with the loss of their ovaries.

Some slowdown in knowledge retrieval does come with age—for both men and women. You know as much or more than you ever did, but it takes longer to recall the information. A friend of ours who competed in the Seniors Tournament on the TV show *Jeopardy!* explained that older contestants score better than younger ones on the preliminary written test. But because older people don't summon the information quite as fast, they're at a disadvantage in the actual game, where speed matters as much as knowledge. Hence the show has created a separate tournament for people over the age of 50. The questions are just as difficult, but the pace is slightly slower.

For your own peace of mind, it's important to distinguish between perimenopausal forgetfulness and the normal slowdown in information retrieval that comes with age. If you're simply one second slower on the office cal-culator than you used to be, don't worry. This is normal, more than offset by your experience, and shouldn't affect your job performance or self-esteem at all. But if your short-term memory seems to have gotten drastically worse, or you can't stay with a simple task like a crossword puzzle, your symptoms may be linked to estrogen withdrawal.

The solution: Face it, we've all known for years that female hormones make you smarter, and now there's proof. There are estrogen receptors found throughout the brain, and estrogen has been shown to influence the growth of nerve cells within the brain. Women who receive HRT report that their ability to remember things improves almost immediately.

Anything that helps you sleep better will help you con-centrate better the next day. Don't hesitate to make lists, to write yourself notes, even to carry a map of your own home-town in the glove compartment if needed. Most importantly, relax. You are not getting dumb or going nuts, and this too shall pass.

Menstrual Irregularity

The problem: The night before you leave on a weeklong business trip your period starts. You set out the next day, equipped with tampons and pads, but by the time you arrive, you've stopped bleeding. You wear a pad the next day as a precaution, and by lunch you're bleeding again, this time quite heavily, with cramps. The bleeding lasts only two days, but you keep using the tampons throughout the trip just in case. When you get home you aren't sure if you should mark the bleeding on your calendar as a period. Who knows when you'll bleed again?

For one woman in 10, periods will simply stop. But for the other 90 percent, the menstrual cycle gradually begins to change.

Unfortunately, there is no way to predict how it will change. Your periods may become shorter, longer, lighter, heavier, closer together, or further apart. Some women who have never experienced cramps begin to have them, and others who have never experienced PMS begin to have all the symptoms.

The solution: For starters, chart your bleeding. The first thing that changes is the length of your menstrual cycle, and unless you have an accurate record of when and how much you're bleeding, hormone replacement therapy can't help.

Progesterone will regulate your periods almost immediately and some HRT regimens stop menstrual bleeding altogether. The pros and cons of these methods will be discussed in the next chapter. Also, if you're still potentially fertile, oral contraceptives will keep your periods regular and prevent pregnancy.

Mood Swings

The problem: The dry cleaner tells you he couldn't get the spot out and you burst into tears.

Although this is one of the symptoms most associated with menopause, research has not proven it to be directly connected. The stereotype of the menopausal women sobbing and raging her way through the day finds little support in clinical studies.

Here's what we do know: Women are two to three times more likely than men to experience depression, but the onset is most often in the late 30s and early 40s, and more often linked to life changes than hormonal changes. The more severe the depression, the less apt it is to be linked to menopause; although some mood swings can be attributed to fluctuations in your hormone levels, most women report just feeling on edge or like "I'm not coping as well as I was"—not suicidal or profoundly unhappy.

So when we speak of menopause "causing" depression, it should be clear that we're talking about moodiness, not complete despair.

Also, the women who report depression in menopause often have a history of psychological disorders. If a woman is teetering on the brink of depression anyway, it's not hard to see how a symptom such as sleep deprivation, memory loss, or having her period every day of the month could quickly become the final straw. Because estrogen and progesterone affect the brain chemicals that regulate appetite as well as sleep and pain perception, variations in hormone levels can lead to corresponding fluctuations in how well you're coping with the most basic requirements of daily life. It's not that estrogen deprivation brings you a whole new set of mental or emotional problems, but it can diminish your capacity to cope with the problems you already have.

The solution: Anything that improves your general health will improve your mental outlook. Try to follow a well-balanced diet and a regular program of exercise, and make sure you get adequate amounts of sleep. HRT can also quickly quell the mood swings that accompany unstable hormone levels, restoring a sense of well-being and calm.

If your depression persists, you feel bad all the time instead of occasionally, or you begin to contemplate suicide, you are not dealing with normal perimenopausal moodiness. You should see your family physician or a mental health professional immediately. Midlife is certainly not too late to make changes, and if your unhappiness is linked to a bad job or bad relationship, a therapist or support group can help you make decisions about your situation. Women in their 40s often feel that they have to be strong for everyone, especially if they're caught between the needs of their still-dependent children and imminently dependent parents. Finding someone to listen, be it a counselor or a group of other midlife women facing similar changes, can make a difference in your outlook.

Perimenopausal moodiness will pass, but true depression does not, and this is another case in which denying the problem will only set you up for a bigger crisis in the future. Many medications can help control anxiety or depression, and these are not the heavily addictive, zombie-making pills that were routinely doled out to the women of our mothers' generation. Better antidepressants, capable of calming you without putting you in a stupor or rendering you unable to make a decision, are available, and you shouldn't hesitate to use them if necessary. Selective serotonin reuptake inhibitors (SSRIs), including medications such as Prozac, Zoloft, Paxil, and Celexa, help you maintain steady levels of serotonin, the "feel-good" nerve transmitter. One word of caution: Just because these drugs are less addictive than antidepressants of the past, don't make the mistake of casually going on and off your medication based on mood, time of year, or changes in the weather. Talk to your doctor and devise a plan for how long you will take the medication and how you will go off of it when the time is right.

Declining Libido

The problem: You wait until you're sure your husband's asleep before you go to bed.

A lack of estrogen leaves the genitals less sensitive to stimulation, so estrogen deprivation alone is enough to damage your libido.

But there's another issue: One of the most interesting and little-known facts about the ovary is that it manufactures small amounts of the male hormone testosterone, which is the libido hormone for both women and men. When its production suddenly stops, either through surgical removal of the ovaries or ovarian failure following chemotherapy, your sex drive can drop. (Testosterone production usually continues for several years after estrogen production has ceased, so a testosterone-related loss of libido in the early stages of natural menopause is unusual.)

Before seeking treatment for low sex drive, consider whether your lack of interest might be a secondary symptom of another condition: Are you exhausted from months of interrupted sleep? Are you depressed, especially about aging issues or your relationship with your partner? Having irregular periods? Most significant, has intercourse become uncomfortable due to vaginal dryness? Anyone will avoid sex if it hurts, and vaginal dryness is a common and treatable symptom of perimenopause.

The solution: Sexuality is complex, and a great illustrator of the mind-body connection. Some women believe, perhaps subconsciously, that age 50 is the automatic end of their sexual selves, and their bodies respond to their minds' grim prediction. The psychology of midlife sexuality will be discussed more in Chapter 10.

Conventional HRT can help reverse declining sexual interest due to falling estrogen levels. If, however, your ovaries have been removed or disabled, HRT can be expanded to include testosterone. This is powerful stuff, so there can be some side effects. But if the dosages are controlled, you should not experience facial hair growth, a lowered voice, or any of the other horror stories you may have heard about. On the plus side, some women report that even with just a little testosterone, they not only get their sex drive back, but they positively feel like they own the street.

Vaginal Dryness

The problem: You and your husband begin to make love. You think you're aroused—or at least you're mentally excited—but you just don't lubricate. Your husband asks, "Is something wrong?" You say no because you expect that once intercourse begins you'll loosen up and lubricate. Instead it hurts, almost as if each thrust is tearing your vagina. After just a few seconds your husband doesn't have to ask if anything's wrong. Something clearly is.

As estrogen levels drop, the vaginal lining thins, the walls become dryer and less elastic, and the vagina itself may actually shorten. Intercourse with inadequate lubrication is often uncomfortable enough to prompt a woman to avoid sex. If the condition remains untreated to the point where the vaginal lining thins or atrophies, intercourse becomes truly painful.

The solution: Vaginal dryness is associated with decreased blood flow to the area, so regular stimulation will keep your vagina more elastic and lubricated. Regular sex and/or masturbation is your first line of defense. If you have a partner, you both need to understand that it may take more foreplay to get you ready for intercourse. Just as your memory retrieval system tends to slow slightly with age, so may your sexual response time, but in both cases the ability is still there. Relax and give yourself time.

If vaginal dryness is your only symptom of perimenopause, you may not require the full HRT package. Vaginal dryness can be treated locally in three ways: lubricants, estrogen replacement cream, or Estring, an estrogen-containing silicone ring that remains in the vagina for three months at a time.

Lubricants make sex more comfortable, but don't address the underlying problem. They are your best bet only if your vaginal dryness is relatively rare. Two popular lubricants are Probe and Astroglide, which can be applied right before intercourse; both are light in texture and have no medicinal taste or smell. Another option is Replens, described as a "vaginal moisturizer," which can be applied hours before intercourse. Replens causes the vagina to retain its natural fluid not unlike an expensive face cream causes the skin to plump up temporarily. If used four times a week as directed, Replens often restores moisture to the degree that an additional lubricant is not needed, and many women prefer it for this reason. Of course, Astroglide and Probe do have far more exciting names.

Estring, the vaginal ring, has the advantage of releasing the estrogen slowly and locally, meaning that very little of the hormone is absorbed into the bloodstream. A woman should expect to see beneficial effects within the first month of use. Like a tampon or diaphragm, a woman does not feel the Estring once it is in place (nor does her partner), and many women appreciate the fact that beyond ring replacements every three months, they don't have to think about the problem.

If your vaginal dryness is chronic or pronounced, your doctor will likely prescribe an estrogen cream or Estring. In comparison to oral estrogen or skin patches, the vaginal creams and rings supply very little estrogen—sufficient to lubricate the vagina but not enough to protect against heart disease and osteoporosis, or to quell hot flashes. But just as the creams and rings provide fewer of estrogen's benefits, they also pose fewer of its risks, and they have the advantage of working rapidly to restore vaginal moisture.

In more severe cases—the vagina has begun to shrink or tear, for example—full-scale HRT will be necessary to restore vaginal function. Unfortunately, it may take several months on oral or transdermal estrogen for the vagina to regain its elasticity and moisture. In the meantime, a topical hormone cream or the Estring can jump-start lubrication and make the idea of sex more appealing. Within a few months your vagina will have begun to respond to the HRT and you'll be able to stop using the cream.

Vaginal dryness has two more bothersome side effects. First, even if sex doesn't actually hurt, a woman in estrogen withdrawal may find that her tissues are less sensitive to stimulation. One woman described this as feeling as if there were an extra layer of skin between her and her partner. Another unwelcome complication is an increased tendency to contract minor vaginal infections. HRT improves both conditions. In addition, if you are prone to vaginal infections, wearing cotton panties, sleeping with no underwear, and avoiding the prolonged use of tampons should help.

Urinary Incontinence

The problem: You sneeze and you wet yourself.

There are two kinds of urinary problems associated with perimenopause, and they have two different solutions. Some women simply lose control, and a small amount of urine is released whenever they laugh, cough, or sneeze, not unlike the common incontinence that follows childbirth. The reason is the same: The muscles in the pelvis have become lax. Ordinarily the pelvic floor supports the bladder, but as it weakens, either due to repeated childbearing or estrogen deprivation, the bladder can drop out of place. Then even the slight pressure of a single cough can trigger a loss of urine.

The second problem is frequent, painful, or urgent urination.

A woman may feel as if she has to urinate all the time, even though her mad dash to the rest room results in only a few drops. The urethra has receptors for estrogen, and without this hormone, the urethra can atrophy much like the vagina. The walls become thinner, weaker, and more susceptible to infection or irritation.

The solution: If your condition is due to slack muscles, you may be able to turn the condition around with Kegel exercises.

Sound familiar? Named after the doctor who developed them, Kegels are the rhythmic exercises that women are sometimes told to do after childbirth to restore muscle tone. A Kegel is simply a tightening and releasing motion, as if you were trying to stop the flow of urine. (In fact, if you have trouble getting the hang of them, you may want to practice by stopping the release of urine while on the toilet, letting it start again, stopping it again, and so on, until you're familiar with what the muscle contraction feels like.)

The Kegel is a small, subtle movement, and the key to success is to do many of them. Begin with 10 and work yourself up to 10 sets of 10. Women who are most successful with Kegels tend to have found a way to work them in to their daily routine: They do them when they're on the phone, in the car, or watching the nightly news. (One woman we interviewed swears she can reach orgasm simply by doing Kegels; if you happen to be this lucky, you may want to rethink doing them while driving.)

Urinary stress incontinence can be persistent, though, and some women need more help. Because urinary tract infections are a frequent side effect of stress incontinence, you should be evaluated and treated for any infections first. Estrogen, especially if administered in the form of vaginal cream, is a direct approach to the problem. HRT will thicken and tone both the vaginal wall and the urethra, while improving the results from your Kegel regimen.

If your pelvic relaxation is too severe to respond to HRT, surgical correction may be necessary. But beware the doctor who advises an operation without giving HRT and Kegels a try; demand a cystometrogram to evaluate your bladder function before agreeing to surgery.

Headaches

The problem: Your head hurts. It feels like a premenstrual migraine—except you get one once a week.

Sometimes rising and falling estrogen levels can cause headaches. Women who were prone to premenstrual migraines are especially likely to experience perimenopausal headaches. HRT can also be a culprit; when women first begin taking HRT, the hormone levels jump rather erratically, resulting in headaches that, although temporary, can be intense.

The solution: If you're on HRT and prone to headaches, consider using the skin patch instead of pills. A more steady absorption of the hormone may prevent the headaches.

Anything that triggered a migraine in your premenopausal days—certain foods, alcohol, poor sleep, or stress—is apt to trigger one now. Regular exercise reduces the number of headaches, and biofeedback has greatly helped many regular migraine sufferers. If all else fails, your physician can subscribe medication specifically for the treatment of migraines.

Joint Aches and Back Pain

The problem: You have a constant dull backache, somewhat like the ones you used to get before your periods would start. Or perhaps you notice a more pronounced ache in your joints and muscles after exercise.

Joint and back pain is an occasional secondary complaint of perimenopause, even among women who do not have a history of joint disease or arthritis.

The solution: Regular exercise helps, especially yoga and stretching, which can maintain and improve joint flexibility. Be sure to learn your moves in a class with a qualified instructor, however. Improperly done, some stretches can cause more injuries than they prevent. Strengthening abdominal muscles through exercises can stabilize your torso and help prevent lower back pain. HRT also helps joint aches, although no one is exactly sure why.

Joint aches can be a fairly inconspicuous complaint. Some women don't realize they suffer from them until they begin HRT and suddenly find it easier to garden or play tennis.

Dry Skin, Wrinkling, and Itching

The problem: Your skin has begun to sag and wrinkle. You feel like you look noticeably older than you did last year.

Skin wrinkling occurs as we age for many reasons, most notably sustained exposure to the sun and the gradual loss of collagen, the protein responsible for the skin's elasticity and tone. Only recently have we begun to fully understand the role estrogen plays in collagen production, but studies have shown that menopausal women on estrogen have thicker skin with a higher collagen content than women who do not take estrogen.

Estrogen also affects the ability of the skin to retain moisture. Any woman who has ever experienced premenstrual bloating can attest to the effect hormones have on fluid retention; women who are treated with high dosages when they first begin HRT also complain of bloating. But mild bloating is a plus for the face: Skin plumped up with moisture looks and feels younger and healthier.

A very small percentage of women experience a problem called formication that makes mere wrinkles seem like a party. Formication is the sensation that bugs are crawling on your skin, a persistent itchiness or tingling sensation that goes far beyond the normal irritation of dry skin. Fortunately, this is a rarely reported symptom, and one that is quite responsive to HRT.

The solution: The two best ways to avoid wrinkles are to stop smoking and stop tanning.

Women's magazines have published numerous articles on good skin care, debating the merits of the numerous collagen-replacement products on the market. Alpha- and beta-hydroxy acid creams are available over the counter and may improve the appearance of the skin. Many moisturizers and cosmetics contain sunscreen, and you should look for an SPF of at least 15.

Some women opt for cosmetic surgery. But many plastic surgeons will not perform a face-lift on a perimenopausal woman who is not on HRT, so vital is estrogen to the healing and health of skin. Surgery can lift the skin back into position, but without the elasticity that comes with adequate estrogen, the long-term benefits of the surgery are lessened and the skin will begin to sag again much more quickly. Although no one is suggesting that you undergo HRT strictly for cosmetic reasons, more youthful skin is an undeniable benefit of hormone replacement.

4

❧

Hormone Replacement Therapy

I'm out of estrogen and I've got a gun.
> —Slogan on a coffee cup

The use of hormone replacement therapy is one of the most complex and controversial aspects of menopause, as reflected in the fact that although 85 percent of doctors advocate HRT, only 20 percent of American women over the age of 50 are currently following their doctors' advice. Why do so few women opt for HRT? Possibly because they have so many unanswered questions: Should you try a therapy that reduces your chance of a heart attack but may increase your risk of breast cancer? How do you wade through all the potential dosing regimens and find the right one for you? Will you still have periods? Is HRT something you do for a couple of years until the hot flashes abate, or is it a decision for life?

For women in perimenopause, hormone therapy is technically a matter of adding estrogen and progesterone, not replacing it, because the ovaries of perimenopausal women are still producing hormones. But because hormone levels vary erratically during perimenopause, additional estrogen and progesterone may be needed to quell the symptoms described in Chapter 3.

In this chapter, we'll look at the benefits and draw-backs of hormone replacement therapy, discuss the most common types of medication, and address the concerns women have about HRT. The goal is neither to preach nor frighten, but to give you enough information to help you enter into an informed discussion with your physician about what's right for you.

Natural vs. Medicated Menopause

For some women, the debate on HRT is over before it begins, because they have a philosophical aversion to med-ical intervention in a natural process. Consider these com-mon protests against HRT:

Argument:
It's not natural.

Rebuttal:
Frankly, it's not natural to live this long. A century ago, dis-eases such as polio and diphtheria wiped out a certain per-centage of the population before it reached adulthood. Childbirth was much more hazardous. Women who made it to menopause were considered elderly, and were not expected to live more than a decade past "the change." But because our generation will on average survive into our 80s, what will happen to the American health-care system if heart disease and osteoporosis incapacitate this huge block of women? Does it make sense to use medicine to extend the length of life but not to improve its quality?

Remember what the "R" in HRT stands for. This ther-apy is not adding something new—it's replacing what the body was once able to produce naturally for itself with a synthetic version. A woman taking estrogen is like a dia-betic taking insulin: She's putting back what was lost, not introducing something completely foreign into her system.

Another point to ponder: If men lost their testosterone at age 50, do you think they'd hesitate to replace it?

Argument:
My mother didn't do it.

Rebuttal:
If you are a typical woman of the baby boomer generation, by this point in your life you have undoubtedly done many things that your mother didn't do.

If your family follows the statistical norm, your mother will not live as long as you will live. An extended life span calls for a different health-care strategy.

It's also possible that your mother defined middle age very differently than you do. Women who are approaching menopause today have high expectations for their energy level and ability to cope with daily life. Your mother may indeed have survived menopause without any intervention, but if her symptoms were severe, the odds are that she simply endured them, figuring that this was just the way women felt after age 50. Today it is less common for women to accept such a "grin and bear it" attitude toward their health.

Argument:
I'm afraid of the side effects—especially the increased risk of cancer.

Rebuttal:
HRT does indeed pose side-effect risks, though there are also risks that come with not taking HRT. Each woman sitting at the table has been dealt a different genetic hand, and she will have to adjust her strategy to fit the particular cards she holds. Look at your family and individual medical history. A woman with a predisposition toward osteoporosis or Alzheimer's disease may make a different decision than a woman with a history of breast disease.

Argument:
It's too complicated.

Rebuttal:
We will grant you this much. HRT is complicated but com-
prehensible. You're already making a start by reading up
on the subject, and the next step is to find a doctor who
will take time to explain your options and address your
concerns.

Since we wrote the first version of this book five years
ago, much more information about menopause has become available to the layperson. The North American
Menopause Society (NAMS) is a group of health-care pro-
fessionals whose annual meetings encompass all aspects of
menopause treatment, from HRT to alternative therapies
such as herbs and soy protein. Physicians who are members of this organization tend to be more eclectic in their
approach to menopause, and may be more open to a dialogue with their patients than more traditional doctors.
The NAMS Web site—www.menopause.org—is an excellent resource and includes links to other areas of interest.
For address and phone information for NAMS, see the
Sources section at the end of this book. (It's a good idea
to keep in mind that the Internet is not foolproof when it
comes to presenting accurate medical information.)

There's plenty of information available, but what still
is lacking—for HRT as well as all the issues of menopause—is a readily accessible support network like the one
that exists for childbirth. When a woman decides she
wants to try delivering her second child vaginally after having the first via cesarean, she's seeking a "VBAC," a vaginal
birth after cesarean. With a few phone calls, she is able to
find a support group, a shelf full of books on the subject,
and a list of physicians and midwives in her area with experience in VBAC delivery. A woman suffering severe vaginal
dryness and atrophy in menopause is certainly in need of
the same support, but it's highly unlikely she'll find any

system in place to help her, much less a group of sympathetic friends and sensitized doctors to see her through the condition.

Argument:
My symptoms aren't that bad.

Rebuttal:
For many women, the symptoms aren't severe and can be handled with the passage of time or the natural remedies outlined in Chapter 5. But even women without severe symptoms should consider the long-term health risks. If you have a family history of heart disease, Alzheimer's, or osteoporosis, HRT is worth investigating, even if you never feel a single hot flash.

Argument:
It's just not me.

Rebuttal:
You'll get no argument from us on this one.

Women must join forces for some purposes: to bring attention to the health-care issues our generation will face as we age, to help make information more readily available, to support the percentage of us who will suffer pronounced distress in perimenopause, and to ensure that more money is spent on research into "women's diseases" such as breast cancer and osteoporosis.

But like all other sexual/reproductive issues, HRT is intensely personal. Just as with an issue like abortion, how you feel about it politically and what you might personally opt to do could well be two different things. As midlife women lobby to be taken seriously by the medical community, we may stand as a group, but when it comes time to take that pill or not take it, each woman stands alone. Try not to base your decision on a certain philosophical agenda. Instead, base it on your personal risk factors, the severity of your symptoms, and your tolerance for physicians, medications, and routines in general.

What Does HRT Do?

HRT effectively treats hot flashes, vaginal dryness, and urinary incontinence. Insomnia and moodiness improve, as does memory and concentration. Periods become lighter and more regular. Freed from these problems, many women report that their energy levels return to normal. Estrogen also does a lot to protect against heart disease, Alzheimer's, and bone loss. There are cosmetic benefits as well; some consider estrogen to be a type of youth drug, producing more elastic skin and shinier hair.

You should seriously consider hormone therapy if:

♦ Menopause is making you miserable. Your symptoms are affecting your quality of life.

♦ Your ovaries have been removed, you've undergone chemotherapy, or for some reason have experienced menopause earlier than is typical.

♦ You have a family history of heart disease or lifestyle factors that put you at high risk for it.

♦ You have a family history of osteoporosis or are at high risk for it.

♦ You have a family history of Alzheimer's.

HRT: A Process of Trial and Error

You'd think that with its list of benefits, women would be stampeding to take estrogen, but in reality only 20 percent of women over 50 are on HRT. Just as significantly, 20 percent of the women who try HRT stop within nine months—and that's probably a lowball figure because many women who don't like HRT simply never return to their physician and, as a result, their experiences are not figured into the statistics. Most of the women who throw in the towel do so because of side effects such as bloating, break-through bleeding, or nausea. A lucky few achieve the perfect combination immediately, but for most women, HRT involves as much as a year of fiddling with the dosage, and several visits to the physician.

Most likely, after trying your first regimen for three months, you'll revisit the doctor to discuss your progress and side effects or complications. At this point, changes may be made in the dosage, the brand of medication, or the method of administration. After you've found a combination that produces either few or no unpleasant side effects, the next visit, scheduled six to nine months after you start HRT, is to see if you are still doing well. At this point you may need further alterations in dosage. The aim of HRT should be to find the most effective dose for each individual woman, low enough to minimize side effects while still high enough to treat her symptoms and protect her from long-term health risks. Eventually, within 18 months, you should have found a combination that works for you.

Even in an ideal scenario, a woman should plan on three to five office visits to regulate her HRT. Some women have to be far more persistent. We interviewed one woman who tried 15 different drugs before she found relief. Obviously, if you're going to be seeing your physician this frequently and putting a good deal of faith in his or her judgment, it's essential to have the right doctor. In Chapter 9 we'll discuss how to find someone who will listen and take the time to fine-tune your particular therapy. If you and your doctor don't have a good rapport, your chances of successful HRT diminish and you're much more likely to become one of the women who give up on it too soon.

How Much Is Enough?

HRT has three goals:

- ♦ to treat acute symptoms such as hot flashes and night sweats
- ♦ to treat intermediate symptoms such as vaginal dryness and urinary incontinence
- ♦ to provide long-term health protection against coronary disease, Alzheimer's, and bone loss

HRT is very individual, and different women will require different types of estrogen, dosages, routes of administration, and length of therapy. In addition, the amount of HRT a woman needs may vary over time; you may function well on a low dose of estrogen for perimenopause, need more when you enter full menopause, and return to a lower "maintenance" dose in your 60s.

Estradiol is the predominant form of estrogen the ovaries produce before menopause, and estradiol levels vary from 40 pg/ml (picogram/milliliter) to 400 pg/ml during a typical menstrual cycle. After menopause, levels fall to 20 pg/ml or less. Generally, a dosage that produces a blood level of 50 to 65 pg/ml of estradiol will relieve symptoms and protect the heart and bones. Some women will require higher levels to feel their best—80 to 120 pg/ml has proven to be a helpful range for women with marked symptoms—but the goal is to use the lowest dose that gets the job done.

Women who had problems with birth control pills sometimes assume that they're not good candidates for HRT, but the dosage of estrogen required to suppress ovulation is three to five times higher than that required to relieve the symptoms of menopause. If you have memories of side effects such as weight gain and bloating on the Pill, don't automatically rule out HRT; lower dosages also mean fewer side effects.

What Are the Risks?

Side effects of taking estrogen include nausea, headaches, and bloating. The dosage and the way the medicine is administered may influence the degree to which you experience the effects. Progesterone, the hormone that brings on your periods, is often a component of HRT and can produce PMS-like symptoms such as fluid retention, moodiness, breast tenderness, and headaches. (see Figure 4.1).

Beyond side effects, there are long-term health risks for some women. HRT can cause hypertension, liver and blood-clotting problems, and may increase your risk of breast cancer (see Figure 4.2). (We'll discuss breast-cancer risk in greater detail in Chapter 6.) You may be a poor candidate for HRT if:

♦ You have been previously diagnosed with breast cancer, or your mother or sister developed the disease before age 50.

♦ You have or have had blood clots or phlebitis.

♦ You have had endometrial cancer.

♦ You have uterine fibroids.

♦ You have had gallbladder or liver disease.

The last two items on the list force a judgment call: Many women with uterine fibroids, or gallbladder or liver disease can still take HRT, but they should be monitored especially closely. Women with liver disease will probably want to opt for the patch method, which allows estrogen to be absorbed directly into the bloodstream, bypassing the liver.

The majority of uterine fibroids—benign tumors common among more than 25 percent of women over 35—do not require treatment; in fact, many women who have fibroids are unaware of it. Sometimes, however, fibroids

Side Effect	Strategy
Bloating	Restrict salt intake, try an herbal diurectic or a mild prescription diuretic, lower the progestogen dose to a level that still protects the uterus, switch to another progestin or natural micronized progesterone.
Weight Gain	Modify diet, exercise to burn calories and fat as well as build up the body's metabolic rate.
Breast Tenderness	Restrict salt intake, lower the estrogen dose, change to another progestin or progesterone, cut down on caffeine.
Headaches	Restrict salt intake, reduce dose of oral estrogen, change to an everyday "continuous" dosage schedule, switch to an estrogen patch.
Depression	Restrict salt intake, change from continuous to cyclic progestin, stop ERT/HRT to see if hormones are the cause.
Nausea	Take estrogen tablets at bedtime or with meals, switch to an estrogen patch.

Figure 4.1 Dealing with ERT/HRT Side Effects

Source: *Menopause Guidebook,* Cleveland, OH: The North American Menopause Society, 1999. Used with permission.

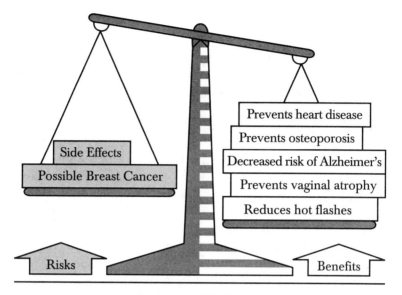

Figure 4.2 Risks vs Benefits of HRT

can cause abdominal discomfort or heavy menstrual bleeding. The standard treatment used to be hysterectomy, but new procedures allow doctors to shrink the fibroids with drugs and remove them surgically, while leaving the uterus intact. For most women, the amount of estrogen in HRT is not enough to affect their fibroids, but some tumors are more sensitive to estrogen than others. The typical treatment is to begin HRT, monitor the fibroids on a regular basis, and discontinue the HRT if they appear to be growing.

How Many Hormones Will I Have to Take?

If you've had a hysterectomy, and thus have no risk of uterine cancer, you can take estrogen alone. Estrogen increases your risk of endometrial cancer, so women who still have a uterus should add progestin or progesterone to their regimen to eliminate this added risk. (Progesterone, the natural hormone, can be difficult to absorb unless prescribed in micronized form; for this reason, the synthetic form is usually prescribed in HRT. In this book, we'll use the word *progesterone* when referring to the natural substance and *progestin* when referring to all drugs that act like progesterone when administered to the body.)

Provera/MPA is the most commonly prescribed progestin; Premarin is the most commonly prescribed estrogen. Many physicians will first try 0.625 mg of Premarin daily and 10 mg of Provera/MPA for the last 10 to 12 days a month, but if this standard dosage doesn't work to relieve your symptoms or causes uncomfortable side effects, don't despair. There are certainly other combinations.

Will I Still Have Periods?

With estrogen alone, there is no period. But when progesterone is combined with estrogen in a menopausal woman's HRT, it encourages her body to mimic the monthly menstrual cycle. Progesterone is the hormone that increases after ovulation to encourage buildup of the endometrium and, ultimately, shedding of the lining as a period.

Depending on how you feel about having a period, there are two basic ways to take the medication: cyclically, which causes periods, or continuously, which keeps you from having a period.

The cyclic method involves taking estrogen daily and progestin or progesterone for 12 to 14 days of the month. At the end of the progestin therapy, you have a period. For many women bleeding is light, somewhat like the periods you have when you're on the Pill. (For some women the bleeding is even lighter, and they eventually get to the point where they don't bleed at all when they stop the progestin.)

In continuous therapy you take lower dosages of progestin—say, 2.5 mg daily of Provera instead of the standard 5 or 10 mg—but you take both the estrogen and progestin every day of month. There are no days off of medication, so no bleeding.

So why doesn't every woman opt to be period-free? The problem with continuous therapy is break-through bleeding, and many women prefer the predictability of the cyclic method to the random bleeding of continuous therapy. If you're willing to persist with the continuous method, however, it's helpful to know that most women manage to overcome the break-through bleeding and totally eliminate all periods within a year.

Dosing Regimens

It's not just what you take, it's also when you take it and what else you're taking with it. HRT encompasses several dosing regimens. We outline some of the most common dosing regimens in the sections that follow.

Continuous Estrogen

If a woman doesn't have a uterus, she can take unopposed estrogen every day of the month, usually in the form of pills or skin patches. Progestin is the component of HRT most likely to cause side effects, so if you don't need it, don't take it.

Cyclic Estrogen Plus Cyclic Progestin

Estrogen is given daily for the first 25 days of the month with progestin added for the last 12 days. (Administration is often adjusted to fit individual needs and the progestin may be required for as few as 10 or as many as 14 days to regulate bleeding.) After the twenty-fifth day, both hormones are stopped and the woman will have a light period. The disadvantage of this program is that symptoms may recur during the five to six days without estrogen.

Continuous Estrogen Plus Cyclic Progestin

Most menopause experts recommend this regimen. A good choice for women with acute symptoms, it involves a daily administration of estrogen, with progestin added for 12 to 14 days of the month. Because you never go off the estrogen, your symptoms never recur, but using the progestin in cyclic dosage means you'll still have a period. Which 12 to 14 days you take the progestin—that is, when you have your period—is up to you, because your period begins as soon as the progestin part of the therapy winds down. If want to avoid always having your period during end-of-the-month holidays such as Thanksgiving and Christmas, start taking your progestin on the first day of the month and your period will begin around the fifteenth day of the month.

For women who take estrogen via the patch, the system is similar. Some brands of the patch last three days, so after you've gone through four patches, begin adding progestin in pill form. Other brands last a week, so you'll add progestin after you've gone through two patches. Whatever brand you use, keep changing the patches throughout the month, because the estrogen is continuous, but discontinue the progestin after 12 to 14 days, and you'll have your period.

Continuous Estrogen Plus Continuous Progestin

This regimen was developed for women who wish to avoid the withdrawal bleeding or periods that begin when you stop taking progestin. Both estrogen and progestin are taken daily, with the progestin or progesterone in a dose lower-than-used cyclicly. As mentioned, women starting out in this regimen commonly experience irregular breakthrough bleeding for six to nine months. But if you can stick it out until you and your doctor fine-tune your progestin dosage, this program usually stops periods altogether within a year.

Continuous estrogen and progestin seem to work best when the regimen is started after a woman has been menopausal for several years or has been on the Pill (with diminishing menstrual flow) in perimenopause. These women are more likely to have little or no menstrual bleeding on this regimen. In contrast, this regimen does not work well for women in the early stages of perimenopause because they tend to bleed all the time.

Continuous Progestin Alone

For women who can't take estrogen, continuous progestin has been shown to relieve hot flashes, and it may prevent bone loss. It has no heart or brain function benefits, however, and doesn't relieve vaginal or urogenital symptoms. Another drawback: The dosage of continuous progestin needed to relieve hot flashes tends to be higher than generally used in HRT and may cause side effects such as bloating and mood swings.

Types of Estrogen

Estrogen comes in two basic forms: synthesized (produced in the laboratory from soy) and "natural" (distilled from horses' urine). Herein lies some of the controversy of what constitutes "natural" estrogen. Maybe a better question is, "What works best for you?"

Premarin

This commonly used form is purified from the urine of pregnant mares, hence the name. Typical doses are 0.625 and 1.25 mg. Higher doses of 2.5 and 5 mg are available but rarely used.

17b-Estradiol

This is the predominant form of estrogen produced by the ovaries before menopause. It is available in both oral (brand name: Estrace) and transdermal forms. Transdermal brand names include Fempatch (which is available only in low doses for perimenopausal "additive" therapy), Alora and Vivelle (which are used twice weekly), and Climara (which is used weekly). The transdermal form initially bypasses the liver; when taken in the oral form, the liver converts 17b-estradiol to estrone (a weaker estrogen) before releasing it into general circulation. The usual dose is 1 to 2 mg taken orally (or 0.05 to 0.1 mg for the patch), but the FDA has approved a smaller oral dosage of 0.5 mg developed solely for prevention of bone loss. A dosage of less than 1 mg orally or 0.05 mg transdermally usually doesn't relieve full-blown symptoms. However, low doses are a good option for postmenopausal women whose symptoms have long since abated and who are taking estrogen only for its long-term health benefits, or for perimenopausal women who are still producing some estrogen on their own.

Estrone Conjugate

This is a derivative of the predominant form of estrogen produced by the postmenopausal ovary, effective for both relieving symptoms and preventing bone loss. Brand names are Ogen and Ortho EST. Some women find they have less menstrual flow on HRT with estrone conjugate than with other forms of estrogen.

Estrone conjugate requires a higher dosage to prevent and treat osteoporosis than Premarin; a form called "esterified estrogen" (brand name: Estratab) is a derivative of soy and has a potency similar to that of Premarin.

Tamoxifen and Other SERMs

Selective estrogen receptor modulators (SERMs) are sometimes called "designer estrogens" because they work as estrogen in some tissues in the body, such as the bones, while working as "anti-estrogens" in other tissues, such as the breasts.

The best known of the SERMs is tamoxifen (brand name: Nolvadex), which is commonly used as an anti-estrogen in the treatment of breast cancer. Tamoxifen does much of the good work of estrogen, such as protecting the bones and heart, but it also poses an increased risk of uterine cancer.

Raloxifene (brand name: Evista), the newest SERM to be approved by the FDA, maintains (but does not rebuild) bones, and acts as an anti-estrogen in the breast without increasing the risk of uterine cancer. Raloxifene's effect on the heart is uncertain; despite lowering cholesterol and LDL (low-density lipoprotein, or "bad" cholesterol) levels in the blood, raloxifene has been shown in one study to be no more effective than a placebo in preventing the build-up of cholesterol in the blood vessels. Nor does it show any beneficial effect on the brain.

Neither tamoxifen nor raloxifene relieve hot flashes, and in fact, they may make the symptom worse. If you are battling pronounced perimenopausal or menopausal symptoms, the SERMs will offer little help; they're more promising for women who wish to offset long-term health risks such as osteoporosis and heart disease without taking a hormone that may increase their risk of breast cancer.

Several new SERMs are currently being tested with the obvious goal of finding a drug that will push all the good estrogen buttons (bone, heart, and brain) while turning off the estrogen effect in the breast and uterus.

Methods of Administration

In the United States today, estrogen can be given via pill, patch, vaginal cream, vaginal ring, or injection. Each method has its pros and cons.

Pills

After being broken down by the intestinal tract and processed by the liver, all oral forms of estrogen essentially produce the same end product, estrone, which circulates in the blood and relieves symptoms. Common brand names of oral estrogen are Premarin, Estrace, Estratab, Ogen, and Ortho EST.

Pluses: Women are often used to taking medication in pill form and it's not hard to make a pill part of your daily routine. The pills are neat and easy to pack when traveling, and, most important, it's simple to alter dosage level if necessary.

Minuses: Estrogens increase the liver's production of clotting factors, which theoretically could place a woman at risk for deep vein thrombosis. This same risk occurs with the Pill—the possibility of blood clots is a major drawback for some women. It's worth remembering, however, that HRT uses a much smaller dosage of estrogen than the Pill does and has a correspondingly lower risk for clotting disorders. Unless you have a personal history of thrombosis or blood clots, this is probably not a problem for you.

In addition, some women develop hypertension on oral estrogens.

Less serious side effects include nausea and bloating. Letting Estrace tablets dissolve under the tongue (rather than swallowing them) may reduce these symptoms while still enabling you to take the medication in pill form. Also, taking estrogen at bedtime seems to put off the sensation of nausea, or at least cause it to occur when you're asleep and unaware.

Patches

Patches containing 17b-estradiol are applied to the skin where they provide relatively constant serum levels. Some of the patches (Estraderm, Alora, Vivelle) are changed every three to four days; others (Fempatch, Climara) are changed weekly. Doses range from 0.025 to 0.1 mg per day.

Pluses: Many women like the patch because once you put it on you can forget about it until it's time to change it. The gradual, constant absorption of estrogen into the bloodstream is effective in muting symptoms and it creates few side effects. Because the patch method bypasses the liver initially, it is a good alternative for women with a history of liver disease. And because the patch doesn't elevate a woman's triglycerides like oral forms of estrogen can, it's a better choice for women at risk for certain lipid disorders and resulting heart disease. As with pills, patches make it easy to change the dosage level if needed.

Minuses: Some women are allergic to the adhesive used to keep the patch on the skin. Other women develop a rash at the site of the patch. Spraying Vancenase (a corticosteroid developed for intranasal use) on the skin prior to applying the patch has been reported to reduce skin irritation. The patch adheres well enough while you're showering or swimming, but may not stay on for prolonged soaks. If you're planning to go hot tubbing or swim the English Channel, you can always remove the patch and put on a new one after your skin dries.

Sweat can also unstick the patch. Women who live in hot, humid climates and athletes who perspire heavily often report that the patches become loosened more readily. Applying paper tape (available in drugstores) in hot weather or when exercising can help hold the patch in place.

Some women do not absorb the estradiol from the patch. If you continue to have menopausal symptoms while on the patch, especially with the larger-dose 0.1 mg patch, you should have your serum estradiol level checked to make sure you're absorbing the estrogen properly.

Occasionally a woman's sexual partner will complain about the aesthetics of the patch, which is generally placed on the hip, thigh, or abdomen. If this is a problem you may want to change your route of administration—or your partner.

Vaginal Creams

Estrogen in cream form can be inserted directly into the vagina, a method that is especially useful in treating vaginal dryness. Don't wait until the situation gets intolerable before seeking help. It takes a long time to overcome a dry or atrophied vagina; even if you're taking HRT in the oral or patch form, it may be necessary to supplement with an estrogen cream to relubricate your vagina.

Vaginal creams are available in Premarin, Ogen, and Estrace preparations. Some estrogen is absorbed through the vaginal lining into the systemic circulation, but the amount of estrogen absorbed isn't enough to prevent heart disease, Alzheimer's, and bone loss. Usually one-quarter of an applicator daily for four weeks is adequate to relieve vaginal dryness, with booster doses a couple of times a week after that. Within a few months, the pill or patch estrogen is enough on its own to alleviate a dry vagina.

Pluses: Creams are by far the quickest treatment of vaginal dryness—the perfect local treatment for a local problem.

Minuses: The creams can be messy, and it's hard to precisely control the dosage. Although there is not enough estrogen in the creams to offer long-term health benefits, sometimes enough is absorbed into the bloodstream to adversely affect other organs, such as the breast or uterus. Thus a woman who experiences side effects from taking estrogen in oral or patch form may find herself developing the same adverse side effects with the creams, although usually to a lesser degree. Also, estrogen cream should not be used directly before intercourse. A man can absorb enough estrogen through his penis over time to cause side effects such as breast enlargement.

Note: A somewhat unusual, but workable alternative for women who don't tolerate oral estrogen or who experience skin irritations from the patch is to insert Estrace tablets into the vagina. The medication is absorbed adequately enough to protect the heart and bones, and the dosage is controlled more easily than with cream preparations.

Vaginal Rings

The vaginal ring (brand name: Estring) is a silicone ring that is inserted into the vagina where it stays for three months. Neither the woman nor her partner can feel it during intercourse. Rings provide very low dosages of estradiol only to the vagina. Because of the low dosage, many physicians feel the Estring can be used to safely treat vaginal dryness or atrophy in patients who have had breast cancer, although it hasn't yet been approved by the FDA for this purpose.

Pluses: The ring can be easily removed if a problem develops. Because of the time-release effect, serum levels of estrogen remain constant as long as the ring is in place.

Minuses: Some women just don't like the idea of "something up there," although one woman we interviewed said the Estring is "like new dental work. You're conscious of it the first couple of days and then you forget about it." Also, women who have had a hysterectomy may have trouble keeping the Estring in place.

Injections

Estradiol preparations can be administered by injection intramuscularly, usually once a month.

Pluses: You don't have to remember to take a pill or replace a patch.

Minuses: You can't remove the medication once it has been injected, even if side effects develop. Also, a woman's tolerance may increase, forcing her physician to prescribe higher doses to achieve the same effect.

On the Horizon: New Methods of Estrogen Administration

These methods of administration are not currently available for use in the United States, but are offered in Europe and may have won FDA approval by the time you need them.

Pellet   Crystalline 17b-estradiol pellets can be implanted under the skin, allowing the estrogen to be absorbed directly into the bloodstream, bypassing the liver. The pellets can remain in place for up to six months until the patient needs another insertion. Insertion of the pellets is a minor surgical procedure, done in the doctor's office under local anesthesia.

Pluses: For six months, you really don't have to think about HRT. Because the estrogen bypasses the liver initially, this is a good option for women with liver problems.

Minuses: The pellets can be difficult to remove if the woman is experiencing side effects. Some women develop a tolerance for the high levels of estradiol in the pellets, necessitating more frequent placement of the pellets and/ or higher dosages.

Skin Creams and Gels   17b-Estradiol gel, popular in France, can be applied to the abdomen and absorbed through the skin. The gel is currently being tested in the United States, but the release date was still unknown at press time.

Pluses: The gels are a no-fuss, noninvasive way to relieve minor symptoms.

Minuses: They're messy to apply and achieving precise dosages is difficult.

Types of Progestin

Although progestin doesn't come in as many forms as estrogen, you still have options.

Natural or "pure" progesterone is poorly absorbed when taken orally, unless taken in micronized form. A new brand, Prometrium, is now available; because it doesn't have to be mixed by individual pharmacists, it ensures more even dosages and better quality control. At least 200 mg, taken cyclically, is usually required to protect the lining of the uterus. Because progesterone makes many women drowsy, 200–300 mg taken before bedtime is a common dosing regimen. The pills or capsules can also be placed directly into the vagina, allowing easy absorption into the pelvic blood supply that leads to the uterus. This method causes fewer side effects because lower dosages are used.

Women today have a few more options when it comes to progesterone, but synthetics (progestins) are still more commonly prescribed. One brand of progestin, Provera, is so popular that "provera" and "progestin" are often used as interchangeable terms. Other brand names for medroxy progesterone acetate (MPA) include Cycrin, Curretab, and Amen. Norethindrone is another oral form of progestin (brand names: Micronor and Nor QD).

Daily Provera dosages range from 2.5 to 10 mg, and the side effects of this bring-on-the-blood hormone, not surprisingly, are similar to premenstrual symptoms—bloating, sore breasts, irritability, and a slight weight gain. You may think your PMS has been reincarnated. (Symptoms seem to be more pronounced with MPA, as compared to progesterone or norethindrone.) The symptoms increase over the course of administration; if you take the hormone for 12 days, you'll have more pronounced symptoms on day 10 than on day one.

Progestin can also be taken in the form of vaginal or rectal suppositories. The suppositories must be used twice daily and are predictably messy. This hormone doesn't work well in injection form—the shots are painful and have to be administered frequently.

The Combipatch, which provides both estradiol and the norethindrone form of progestin, recently became available. It releases 0.05 mg of estradiol per day and either 0.14 mg or 0.24 mg of norethindrone, depending upon which patch is prescribed. It can be used either cyclically in combination with an estradiol-only patch or in continuous-combined fashion. The Combipatch is changed twice weekly.

There is also a new progesterone vaginal cream, Crinone, which can be used two or three times a week to protect the endometrium. Using Crinone in menopause is not that common yet, and, like all the cream forms, it can be messy. But, it may be a viable choice for women who cannot tolerate oral or transdermal forms of progesterone.

Testosterone Replacement

In addition to estrogen and progesterone, the premeno-pausal ovaries produce androgens, a group of "male" hor-mones that includes testosterone. In fact, the ovaries continue to produce small amounts of testosterone even after estrogen and progesterone production have shut down, but because these levels are not as high as they are before menopause it makes sense that some women might benefit from androgen replacement.

Testosterone not only boosts the libido but also de-creases the anxiety and mild depression some women suf-fer in perimenopause. Women whose ovaries are removed prior to menopause particularly benefit from testosterone replacement, because the sudden withdrawal of hor-mones often leads to an equally sudden drop in their sex drive. If such a woman is given estrogen, her hot flashes and night sweats may disappear, but she often complains that "something" is still missing. Testosterone replacement turns the lights back on, increasing energy, libido, and general optimism.

Furthermore, testosterone reduces breast tenderness for women who recently began HRT and perimenopausal women who suffer this symptom before menstruation. As an added bonus, testosterone also helps prevent bone loss.

But many women worry about the side effects. Al-though some women experience mild acne and a degree of hair growth, testosterone dosage levels are quite low and very few women report overtly masculine changes such as a deeper voice or noticeable facial hair. Some physicians have speculated that the use of testosterone in women could cause their LDL ("bad" cholesterol) levels to rise and their HDL (high-density lipoprotein, or "good" cholesterol) to fall, increasing their risk of heart disease. But studies of women who take supplemental testosterone haven't shown the hormone to have an adverse effect on their cholesterol levels.

Testosterone can be administered either by injection, pill, or cream. The injection, testosterone enanthate (brand name: Delatestryl), is given every four to six weeks. The pill (brand name: Estratest), combines estrogen and testosterone and can be taken every day or alternated with estrogen every other day, depending upon whether the woman develops any side effects. Halotestin, a synthetic derivative of testosterone, is also used in low doses in HRT.

Testosterone creams are being used more and more. They have even been featured on Oprah Winfrey's show. The woman applies a small amount to her genitals and clitoris. (Although one pharmacist we spoke to suggested applying it on the inside of the arm. Perhaps he knows something we don't.) The worst that can happen is that it won't work or that it will produce mild side effects like minor acne or facial hair. The best that can happen is reflected in the claims of one woman we talked to who became so sexually "energized" she had to send her husband out for Viagra just so he could keep up with her. It's always possible, of course, that a placebo effect is taking place—most women don't respond quite so dramatically to the cream—but as long as she's enjoying herself, does it matter?

On the Horizon: Tibolone, the Combination Pill

Tibolone, a synthetic steroid with the properties of estrogen, progestin, and androgen, is currently being tested in the United States. It has been tested in Europe for more than 15 years and is approved for use in several European countries. With its estrogenic properties, it relieves menopausal symptoms and helps prevent bone loss, while the progestogenic and androgenic properties protect the uterus. However, it is not known whether Tibolone increases a woman's risk of breast cancer, and it seems to offer fewer coronary benefits than HRT.

Tibolone is not a naturally-occurring hormone, and thus is not a good choice for women who want to keep their treatment as natural as possible; in other words, it's a treatment and not a replacement. But for women with a low risk of heart disease, the idea of taking one medication to provide all three of the major components of HRT is undeniably attractive.

The Pill

If the complexities of the previous sections have left you reeling, there's a simpler solution that works for many perimenopausal women.

Are you already on the Pill? Keep taking it.

Today's low-dosage birth control pills, which use only 20 micrograms of ethinyl estradiol, not only prevent pregnancy and keep periods regular but can also reduce perimenopausal symptoms. One brand, Mircette, is particularly interesting because it provides an ultra-low dose (10 micrograms) of estradiol for the week that a woman is having her period. Other birth control pills just provide a placebo—inactive pills—for the week of your period, meaning that a woman with perimenopausal symptoms may regain her hot flashes and night sweats during that week. Mircette can help avoid that. If you're on another brand of the Pill, you can also prevent the return of perimenopausal symptoms by using a low-dose estrogen patch during the week of your period.

Another advantage of using birth control pills through your 40s: If a woman develops a very light menstrual flow on the Pill, she can probably switch to a continuous-combined regimen earlier in menopause and avoid further bleeding.

Note: Ultra low-dose birth control pills are being developed specifically for use in menopause. When they're available, these new Pills with an ethinyl estradiol dosage of 10 to 15 micrograms should offer a convenient, low-risk HRT option.

Is HRT Forever?

How long a woman should take HRT depends upon her goals for therapy. If relief of hot flashes and night sweats is her primary concern, she may need to take HRT for only a couple years, after which she can gradually wean herself from the medication. Vaginal dryness and atrophy usually require longer treatment, but in general a woman using HRT to relieve her menopausal symptoms stays on the medication for two to four years. Dosage can also change through the years: A woman in her 60s may not need as much estrogen as she did in her early 50s when her hot flashes were severe.

Although dosages can be lowered once the symptoms have passed, a woman at high risk for heart disease or osteoporosis may consider staying on estrogen for life. The moment a woman stops HRT, bone loss will resume at the same accelerated rate typical of menopause. Less is known about the prevention of heart disease, but women who have been on estrogen for 10 years or longer have markedly less heart disease than women who took estrogen for only a short time.

But how long to stay on HRT is not a decision you have to make going in. Each year, you and your physician should review the reasons you're on HRT—just as you would do for medications for high blood pressure or diabetes. Reevaluate your symptoms, your response to treatment, any side effects, and your overall health. Both you and your physician should be flexible in your approach, not only as to whether or not to use HRT, but also when determining how long to continue it.

5

Natural Remedies for Menopausal Symptoms

The best way to have a good idea is to have lots of ideas.

—Linus Pauling

In the United States, alternative medicine has moved from the shadows to the limelight. More than one-third of adults take dietary supplements, including vitamins and minerals, herbs, hormones, and amino acids.

Women choose alternative or natural remedies to treat perimenopausal symptoms for lots of reasons. Their doctors may be patronizing or unresponsive to their needs. Symptoms in perimenopause tend to come and go in unpredictable patterns, and several women told us that each time they made a doctor's appointment the troublesome symptoms would mysteriously abate. Furthermore, rubbing yam cream on your abdomen may seem like a simpler, less invasive treatment than full-throttle HRT and more appropriate for a symptom that appears for only a few days each month. Some women cite philosophical reasons for taking the alternative path, such as desire for greater control over their health care or determination not to fool with Mother Nature.

Herbal and dietary supplements are much less strictly regulated than pharmaceuticals, with fewer manufacturers' guidelines to ensure that a particular pill contains what it claims to contain. Europe is ahead of the United States in this area. In Germany, for example, physicians prescribe herbs through pharmacies, and the government has sanctioned as drugs certain herbs that have a track record of safety and effectiveness. American physicians, in contrast, have very little training in the use of herbs and tend to know about only those medications that have shown to be effective in clinical trials. Because of this lack of training, very few American doctors feel comfortable in recommending herbs.

In a double-blind clinical trial, subjects are selected based on age, gender, medical history, and general physical condition. One subject is given the drug or herb being studied and the other is given a placebo, without the patient or doctor knowing which is which. For example, in a clinical trial dong quai, an herb believed to help menopausal women, proved no better than a placebo in relieving hot flashes. That would seem to be the end of it, but here's the rub: The placebo worked in 25 to 40 percent of the cases, as did the dong quai. So, many women reason that if picking up a bottle of dong quai at the local health food store saves them a trip to the doctor and an expensive, and complicated treatment, why not give it a try? If it doesn't work, or, as some women report, it works for only a while and then loses its effectiveness, they can always switch to more traditional treatments later.

Doctors are becoming a bit more savvy about alternative treatments. In late 1998, the *Physician's Desk Reference*, the standard guide to drug use, issued a volume on dietary supplements, and the American Botanical Council has just published a translation of the German Commission E monographs, the official documents used by the German Federal Health agency to regulate the use of herbs. Such publications should help U.S. physicians better understand herbal remedies, and perhaps make them more likely to suggest alternative treatments to their patients— or at least be more accepting of their patients' decisions to use them.

Supplements for treating perimenopausal symptoms fall into three basic categories: nutritional, herbal, and hormonal. Some have good track records of reducing menopausal symptoms, some have proven in studies to render mixed results, and others have either been shown to be ineffective or have a prohibitive risk of side effects.

Nutritional Supplements

Nutrients, such as vitamins and minerals, are normally acquired through the foods in your diet. Nutritional supplements become necessary when you're either not getting enough nutrients in your diet or when higher amounts than typically found in your diet may be beneficial.

Soy

The alternative to HRT that is getting the most attention lately is soybean/isoflavone supplementation. Much of the interest in soy stems from data from the Far East, where the typical diet is high in soy, and rates of heart disease, cancer, and hip fractures are lower than in the West. The rate of reported menopausal symptoms is also lower in Asian women, a statistic that could be attributed to a culture that raises women to "Never complain, never explain," genetics, or something in the eastern lifestyle or diet. It has been noted that when Asian women move to the West and assume a western diet (along with western stress levels), their cancer and heart disease risks approach that of women in their adopted country. This lends credence to the theory that the eastern diet, including soy, is responsible at least in part for eastern women's overall health.

Soy can be thought of as nature's SERM, because it appears to act somewhat like estrogen in the cardiovascular system and bones, and as an anti-estrogen in the breast. Soy protein in a dosage of 45 grams daily has been found to reduce hot flashes by 40 percent (remember that placebos reduce hot flashes by 25 to 40 percent too), and may also benefit the surface cells of the vagina. Many studies have shown that soy also has a positive effect on total cholesterol, LDL ("bad") cholesterol, and triglycerides.

The recommended daily consumption is 45 grams, or close to a quart of soy milk or a pound of tofu. Not your idea of a great lunch? Then try soy supplements such as Take Care, Genisoy, or Revival, which provide about 24 grams per dose, and also supplement with 500 mg of calcium. Some of these products are flavored with chocolate or vanilla to be mixed with milk, juice, or water; others come in the form of energy bars.

Soy is also reported to retard the growth of breast tumors; so far this effect has been studied only in rats, but it is considered a promising area of research, especially considering the fact that Asian women have a lower instance of breast cancer than western women do. Soy has also slowed bone loss in rats. More studies are underway to test soy's effect on human bones.

Red clover blossoms (sold under the brand name Promensil) are also a natural source for the same phytoestrogens (isoflavones) found in soy. The recommended dose per day is 40 mg.

Flaxseed

One study found that flaxseed (also known as linseed) can reduce hot flashes. The study authors suggested using 10 grams of flaxseed daily in combination with tofu. Flaxseed offers antioxidant effects as well as some of the benefits of estrogen, although to a lesser degree. It can be ground in a coffee grinder or food processor and added to breads, muffins, and pizza dough.

Vitamin E

It has become increasingly accepted that vitamin E can reduce the risk of heart disease. In addition to being a valuable antioxidant, some vitamin E devotees believe that vitamin E helps to relieve hot flashes, although there is as yet little evidence that it really works.

The difference between using vitamin E as a nutritional supplement and using it as a natural remedy lies in the dosage.

Although the daily requirement of vitamin E is only about 10 IU daily, when used to reduce heart disease risk or menopausal symptoms it is usually taken at a dose of 100 to 800 IU daily.

However, keep in mind that vitamin E slightly "thins" the blood, so it shouldn't be combined with blood thinners such as Coumadin (warfarin), heparin, Trental (pentoxyfilline) or even aspirin, garlic, or gingko (which also have anticoagulant effects) except under medical supervision.

Omega-3 Fatty Acids

Another nutritional supplement thought to reduce cardiovascular disease is omega-3 fatty acids, or "fish oils" found in cold-water fish. Obviously, the easiest way to introduce more omega-3 into your body is just to eat more of this type of fish. One study reported that a daily 3-ounce serving of salmon, cod, mackerel, haddock, or other cold water fish could reduce a woman's risk of cardiac arrest by 50 to 70 percent. If you don't like seafood, fish oil supplements are available; look for eicosapentaenoic acid (EPA) and docosahexaenoic acid (DHA) on the label. One note: Omega-3 fatty acids might affect blood clotting, so if you take a lot of aspirin or are on an anticoagulant such as Coumadin (warfarin) or heparin, consult your physician before starting omega-3 supplements.

Herbal Supplements

The use of herbal supplements involves using plants as medicine. Don't be misled—herbs are drugs, albeit drugs in a natural form. Herbal medicinal products (marketed in the United States as "dietary supplements") are those with active ingredients exclusively of plant material or vegetable drug preparations. Some of them may be powders, extracts, tinctures, or expressed plant juices, not necessarily the entire plant.

Black Cohosh (Cimicifuga Racemosa)

Tested and widely used in Germany, black cohosh appears to reduce many symptoms of menopause, including hot flashes, insomnia, and depression, with a remarkable 90 percent of patients responding positively within six months in some studies. Early research indicated that black cohosh produces estrogen-like effects on cells in the vagina and uterus, but the most recent evidence suggests that black cohosh does not act as a phytoestrogen. Virtually all scientific studies of black cohosh have used the German product Remifemin, which is also widely available in the United States. This product has strong quality control and a proven track record, but there's no guarantee that other products containing black cohosh on the shelves of your local natural food store will perform as well. Consult a health-care practitioner or herbalist before taking black cohosh.

There are some questions about what constitutes a safe dosage. Ideally, the product should state that it contains 27-deoxyacteine; the proper dose is 2 to 4 mg of deoxyacteine per day.

Germany's Commission E recommends not using black cohosh for more than six months, due to the lack of information about long-term safety. For example, long-term safety with regard to the breast and uterus are unknown.

Dong Quai

By itself, the herb dong quai does not appear to be effective for treating menopausal symptoms. In fact, dong quai has been found in one study to be no better than a placebo in treating menopausal hot flashes. However, traditionally it is usually used in complex herbal formulations rather than alone. These combinations have not been studied in proper scientific trials, but they have been used in China for thousands of years and are thought to be effective. By itself, dong quai can cause increased sensitivity to the sun and, occasionally, fevers. Seldom, however, has it been known to cause any other obvious side effects.

St. John's Wort (Hypericum)

Shown to be effective in treating mild to moderate depression, St. John's wort has become exceedingly popular in the United States. The recommended dose is 300 mg three times daily of an extract standardized to contain either .3 percent hypericin or 3 to 5 percent hyperforin.

St. John's wort is probably not very effective for severe depression. It should not be taken in combination with prescription antidepressants such as Prozac because taking the herb and drug together enhances side effects such as dizziness and headaches. At twice the recommended dosage, St. John's wort can slightly increase sensitivity to the sun.

Ginkgo Biloba

The most popular herb in Europe, ginkgo biloba improves blood flow in the brain and extremities. In the United States it is often promoted as a "smart pill"—and, amusingly, it is given as a consolation prize on the game show "Jeopardy!" The Germany's Commission E indicates that ginkgo can help improve memory and mental function in those with Alzheimer's disease or similar forms of dementia, but we don't know if it helps ordinary age-related memory loss.

The recommended dosage is 120 to 240 mg daily of an extract standardized to contain 24 percent flavonol glycosides and 6 percent terpene lactones. Ginkgo biloba is widely available under many brand names. Ginkgo "thins" the blood and should not be taken prior to surgery, or combined with drugs that also thin the blood, such as Coumadin (warfarin), heparin, Trental (pentoxifylline), or even aspirin.

Mexican Yam

Wild Mexican yams are sometimes billed as "natural progesterone." Mexican yam plus progesterone is available in pill, suppository, and cream form, which is the most common. Although components of the Mexican yam are used in laboratories to synthesize steroid hormones, including estrogen and progesterone, the yam itself doesn't contain hormones or any hormonally active substances

Despite the fact that testing has produced little evidence that Mexican yams help treat the symptoms of menopause, the "yam scam" has become big business. Remember: Unless the cream has been spiked with a hormone such as progesterone, its effects are nil.

Valerian

Valerian is an herbal sedative shown to be effective in relieving insomnia. The usual dosage is 2 to 3 grams taken one hour before bedtime. It seems to take a few weeks of constant use to reach its full effects.

Note: Valerian should not be combined with prescription sedatives. There has been some recent concern about withdrawal symptoms in patients who have taken Valerian over prolonged periods of time. Use caution with any sedative, pharmaceutical or herbal.

Garlic

The theory persists that garlic protects against cardiovascular disease by lowering cholesterol. The claim may be related to the fact that garlic is heavily used in Mediterranean diets and the incidence of heart disease in that region is low.

Two recent studies, however, have not found any benefit with the most common form of garlic, so the picture has become more confused.

In any case, garlic appears to be reasonably safe. The usual dose is one to two cloves of raw garlic daily or

900 mg of garlic powder standardized to contain 1.3 percent alliin. We don't know if cooked garlic is just as beneficial, and garlic oil definitely does not work.

Like ginkgo, garlic can "thin" the blood, so all the same precautions apply.

Kava

Used to treat mild anxiety, some brands advertise on the box that they are specially formulated for "menopausal anxiety," whatever that is. Kava is very popular in Europe, and several studies have shown that it controls anxiety better than a placebo, probably because it affects the same brain chemicals that respond to drugs in the Valium family. The daily dose of kava should supply 140 to 210 mg of the presumed active ingredients called "kavalactones."

Excessive doses of kava can cause a yellow discoloration of the skin, hair, and nails, but this does not occur at normal doses. The most serious potential problem is the risk of coma if you combine kava with other sedative drugs (alcohol, barbituates, and medications in the Valium family). Although kava by itself usually doesn't impair reaction time or mental function, it does make some people drowsy, so don't drive after taking it until you know how it affects you.

Germany's Commission E recommends not using kava for more than 3 months, due to lack of evidence regarding long-term safety.

Ginseng

The Chinese and Koreans have sworn by ginseng for centuries, claiming that it promotes mental and physical vigor. Some people claim that ginseng can help reduce hot flashes for perimenopausal women, but this is not its traditional use. In terms of ginseng's success as a general energizer, the German Commission E recommends it for "invigoration and fortification in times of fatigue, for declining capacity for work and concentration." Makes you want to take some right now!

Ginseng appears to be quite safe when used at typical dosages. However, there are reports of ginseng interacting with certain drugs, including digoxin, anticoagulants, and medications in the MAO inhibitor family. (The last of these may have been due to contaminants in the product, specifically caffeine.)

Hormonal Supplements

Hormones are substances produced by the endocrine glands in the human body and secreted directly into the bloodstream. If your production of these hormones is low or a larger amount might be beneficial, supplements may be needed.

Melatonin

Melatonin, a hormone made by the pineal gland in the human brain, has been billed as the perfect anti-aging pill, as well as a sleep aid and antioxidant. Only the sleep aid claims have been verified. Good evidence tells us that melatonin is effective for jet lag, and it may be helpful for other forms of insomnia as well. The typical dosage is 1 to 3 mg at bedtime to help you fall asleep faster and achieve better rest. However, keep in mind that melatonin is a hormone. We don't really know if it is safe to take it long term. Studies have shown that melatonin causes blood vessels in the brains of rats to constrict, a worrisome side effect, although the same studies have not been done on humans. Other potential drawbacks include confusion,

Acupuncture

Calming and nearly painless for most people, acupuncture involves the placement of very thin needles into various parts of the body to unblock the channels carrying the body's "chi," or life force. According to traditional Chinese medical theory, in this balanced state the body begins to heal itself. Acupuncture is widely thought to be helpful for stress, insomnia, menopausal symptoms and menstrual irregularity, although the level of scientific evidence is not great. It is gaining acceptance among western-trained doctors, some of whom are trained to practice acupuncture themselves.

Needless to say, this is not a do-it-yourself therapy. Most states offer specific licensure for trained acupuncturists. For more information, contact the National Certification Commission for Acupuncture and Oriental Medicine on the Internet at www.nccaom.org.

drowsiness, and morning-after headaches. Also be careful about when you take it: Melatonin taken during the day can disrupt the natural sleep/wake cycle, creating more problems than it solves.

DHEA

A hormone produced in the adrenal gland, DHEA levels naturally decrease with age. Supplemental DHEA has been shown to increase muscle mass in men. DHEA can cause hair growth and might increase the risk of liver cancer. No more than 25 to 50 mg per day of DHEA are recommended. Its benefits are not at all clear.

More information on the natural approach to treating menopausal symptoms is available every day. Magazines such as *Shape, Health, Cooking Light, Self,* and *New Woman* feature regular articles on the topic.

Lowering your general stress level and eliminating toxic substances like nicotine and caffeine are two more ways you can help relieve perimenopausal symptoms and improve your overall health. Consult Chapter 8 for information on stress-reduction techniques and detoxification.

A Symptom-by-Symptom Guide to Natural Remedies

Hot Flashes

1. Try to isolate your "trigger foods," such as coffee, sugar, alcohol, or spicy foods, and then avoid them.

2. Get regular aerobic exercise.

3. Helpful vitamin supplements include vitamin E, vitamin C, calcium, and selenium.

4. Black cohosh and soy protein appear to be helpful supplements as well.

Vaginal Dryness

1. Use over-the-counter lubricants such as Astroglide, Probe, Replens, Moist Again, Gyne-Moistrin, Lubrin, or Today.

2. Remember the use-it-or-lose-it rule: Regular sex and/or masturbation help prevent atrophy.

Insomnia or Night Sweats

1. Set up a regular sleep routine. Go to bed at the same time every night. Avoid insomnia-producing

foods and beverages such as coffee, chocolate, and spicy dishes.

2. Exercise regularly—but not just before bedtime.

3. Use a soothing ritual—a hot bath, a massage, relaxation tapes, or a few yoga postures—to get you in the mood for sleep.

4. Avoid cigarettes and alcohol, both of which can disrupt your sleep cycle.

5. Helpful supplements include melatonin and valerian.

Osteoporosis

1. Do weight-bearing aerobic exercises (such as walking) and weight resistance exercises (such as pumping iron) on a regular basis.

2. Take calcium supplements in the form of calcium carbonate or calcium with magnesium.

3. Eat calcium-rich foods such as milk, yogurt, cheese, and green leafy vegetables.

4. Have a baseline dual energy X-ray absorptiometry (DEXA) exam when you are still in your 40s, then have regular follow-ups to make sure that you're maintaining bone density.

5. Soy protein supplements may be helpful.

Heart Disease

1. Eat a diet high in nutrients and fiber and low in fat. Have your cholesterol checked on a regular basis.

2. Soy protein may help lower a mildly elevated cholesterol level.

3. Do aerobic exercise at least three times a week, keeping your heart rate in its target range for at least 30 minutes each time.

4. Maintain a body mass index (BMI) of 26 or less.

5. Don't smoke.

6. Drink only in moderation.

6

❧

Risky Business: Heart Disease, Osteoporosis, Alzheimer's, and Breast Cancer

Do not take life too seriously. You will never get out of it alive.
—Elbert Hubbard

You may not believe it while you're in the middle of a hot flash, but the symptoms of perimenopause can be your best friends. We all nod sagely when the local newscast runs a special on making lifestyle changes to prevent illness, but human nature being what it is, we are often far less motivated by the threat of the serious health problem 20 years away than we are by the immediate discomfort of the symptom at hand.

Hot flashes and irregular bleeding are the irritants that drive women to their doctors' offices and force them to confront the long-term effects of menopause. Perimenopause can serve as the wake-up call that impels a woman to make the changes she's been talking about making for decades. Although we may not be thrilled when the alarm goes off, we're actually lucky to have a built-in hormonal impetus to get us moving. The wake-up call for men is usually a heart attack.

The four major diseases facing women as they age are heart disease, osteoporosis, cancer, and Alzheimer's disease. Hormone replacement therapy reduces a woman's risk for heart disease, Alzheimer's, and bone loss, but may increase her risk for cancer, especially breast cancer. In a perfect world, all would be clear and the same health plan would work for everyone, but it seems that once hormones enter the picture, nothing is ever perfectly clear again. "What finally makes up your mind about estrogen," said one woman we interviewed, "comes down to what disease you most fear." Let's look at each of the big health fears women face as they age and examine how the conventional means of treatment affects a woman's risk for each.

Heart Disease

The problem: Heart disease is the number one killer of women over 50, who, in fact, have twice as high a chance of dying of heart disease as they do of any kind of cancer. But because the medical community sometimes considers heart attacks to be a male problem, coronary disease in women is under-researched and under-diagnosed.

Estrogen protects women from the hardening of the arteries that precedes many kinds of heart disease, and during the years in which this hormone is in our system, we have a much slimmer chance of heart attack than men do. But when estrogen drops off or disappears, our risk of cardiovascular disease rises sharply.

Women are less likely to be diagnosed and treated for heart disease, partly because they develop it later than men do. The majority of the large federally funded stud-

Risk Factors for Heart Disease

1. Do you have hypertension?
2. Do you have a family history of heart disease?
3. Are you obese? (Obesity is defined as having a body mass index of 30 or higher. A BMI of 26 or higher classifies you as overweight. See the formula for measuring your BMI on page 133.)
4. Do you have a sedentary lifestyle?
5. Do you smoke?
6. Are you under a lot of stress?
7. Are you diabetic?
8. Do you have high total cholesterol, high LDL cholesterol, low HDL cholesterol, or elevated triglycerides? (A simple blood test can tell you how you stand.)

ies on heart disease have been conducted in Veterans Administration hospitals and thus have primarily used male subjects. For every woman who has participated in a heart disease study, thousands of men have been tested, so the treatment of women is generally based on what works for men, with little more than an educated guess as to how female physiology and hormones alter the equation.

Doctors are still more likely to diagnose a woman's chest pains and difficulty breathing as an anxiety attack, not a heart attack, especially if the women is under 50. Most disturbing of all, women die more frequently during coronary surgery than men do. This is not because we're weaker—in general women recover better from surgery—but rather because our heart disease is less likely to be caught in the early stages. By the time a woman ends up in the operating room, she is apt to be a decade older than the man down the hall receiving the same surgery, and her disease is likely to be further advanced. Moreover, women have smaller arteries and veins than men do, so many bypass procedures, which were developed for male patients, don't work as well on women.

The solution: Study after study has shown that estrogen protects the heart. There are two kinds of cholesterol, the "bad" LDL, which carries fat to the blood vessel walls and causes blocked arteries, and the "good" HDL, which carries fat away from the blood vessel walls to the liver, where it is subsequently eliminated. Estrogen works to keep HDL levels high; when estrogen levels decrease, LDL rises sharply. When lost estrogen is replaced, a healthy balance between HDL and LDL is restored.

Of course, simply going on HRT is not the only way you can decrease your chance of heart disease. You should also:

♦ Make sure that less than 30 percent of your daily calorie intake comes from fat.

♦ Exercise aerobically at least three times a week.

♦ Stop smoking immediately, and avoid secondhand smoke.

♦ Stay within an appropriate weight range for your height and frame.

If you have a genetic history and/or lifestyle that predisposes you to coronary problems, or if you have a complicating condition such as diabetes or hypertension, you should educate yourself about what you can do to lower your risk. Making the lifestyle changes we recommend in Chapters 7 and 8 is a good start, but if you have a serious family or personal history of heart disease, you and your doctor should discuss an individualized health-care program that includes close monitoring.

The bad news is that heart disease is rampant. More than half a million people die every year in the United States from heart attacks, and 50 percent of them are women. Although women tend to worry more about breast cancer, five times as many women die each year from coronary disease. The good news is that we can do much to lower our personal risks, beginning with replacing the female hormones that protect our hearts in the years before menopause.

Osteoporosis

The problem: The problem is that you don't know there is a problem. Osteoporosis frequently goes undiagnosed until the age of 70, when you fall and break a hip. Or, more likely, you break a hip first and then fall.

Skipped periods or night sweats are irritating, but osteoporosis is long term and debilitating. During perimenopause, a woman may lose 1 to 1.5 percent of her total bone mass each year. After menopause, bone loss accelerates to an average of 3 percent a year, with some women losing an astounding 6 percent a year. As the bones become thinner, they snap more easily, resulting in breaks from the most minor movements, such as stepping off a curb. Women in the advanced stages of osteoporosis may break bones by merely coughing or rolling over in bed. The back vertebrae, wrists, and hips are the most likely bones to break.

There is a genetic link in osteoporosis, so if your mother or grandmother experienced bone fractures, became noticeably shorter as she aged, or developed the hump back that frequently comes with the disease, consider yourself at higher-than-average risk. In general, small, frail, fair-skinned Caucasian or Asian women are more prone to the disease than tall, big-boned, or black women. Lifestyle choices can also raise your risk. If you have insufficient calcium in your diet, smoke, drink more than two alcoholic beverages a day, or don't exercise, you've already begun to undermine the strength of your skeletal system.

A woman who enters perimenopause with lighter-than-average bones is the proverbial accident waiting to happen. Once the estrogen fluctuations during perimenopause begin, her risk doubles because she's not only prone to losing bone mass faster than a woman in better health but she has weaker bones to begin with. Women who go through menopause by age 45, whether naturally or through surgery or chemotherapy, are also at increased risk, simply because they've had fewer years in which to build up their bones and more years in which their bones are eroding.

How prevalent is osteoporosis? Twenty-five percent of Caucasian and Asian women will develop a spinal compression fracture by age 60—the gradual breaking down of the vertebrae of the spinal column that causes the bones to literally collapse upon each other. Women with this condition become shorter, develop a hump on their backs, and are on track for major spinal problems and pain as they continue to age. Women lose an average of 2.5 inches in height between menopause and age 80.

Other bone fractures follow. Femur and wrist fractures occur around age 70 and by age 80, 20 percent of American women will break a hip. Recovery from a hip fracture is slow, painful, and often incomplete, with a full 50 percent of hip-replacement patients never again able to live on their own. Twenty percent of hip fracture patients die within three months of the accident. Heavy doses of pain medication are frequently required, sometimes causing these elderly women to become permanently confused. It's hard to understand why more attention isn't paid to this largely avoidable disease, which causes so many women to experience chronic pain, use walkers, and live in nursing homes.

Risk Factors for Osteoporosis

1. Did you experience menopause before age 45?
2. Do you have a family history of osteoporosis?
3. Are you thinner than average? Small boned?
4. Do you have or have you ever had low calcium intake?
5. Are you Caucasian or Asian?
6. Have you ever been anorexic? Did your periods ever stop for an extended length of time due to an eating disorder or excessive exercise?
7. Do you smoke?
8. Do you drink more than two alcoholic beverages per day?
9. Do you drink more than two caffeinated beverages per day?
10. Do you fail to exercise on a regular basis?
11. Do you take an anticonvulsant or glucocorticoid on a regular basis?
12. Do you suffer from any of the following medical conditions: menstrual irregularities, hyperthyroidism, Cushing's disease, chronic renal failure, or hypogonadism?

The solution: Part of the reason osteoporosis isn't mentioned more often is that it can be asymptomatic until the moment a bone breaks. Because 25 percent of bone mass can be lost before it shows up on a routine X ray, most of the women who are in the early stages of osteoporosis don't know it. If you have several of the risk factors outlined in this section, you should consider having your bones evaluated prior to menopause.

Healthy bone is visibly denser than bone that has been ravaged by osteoporosis (See Figures 6.1 and 6.2). A dual

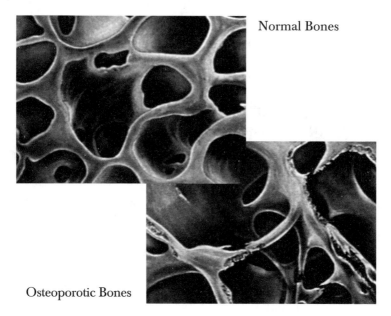

Normal Bones

Osteoporotic Bones

Figure 6.1 X ray of normal and osteoporotic bones.

energy X-ray absorptiometry (DEXA) can better detect early bone loss than a standard X ray. Available at most hospitals as well as many clinics and satellite facilities, a DEXA is a relatively quick, low-dosage radiation technique used to measure a woman's overall bone density and to evaluate the lumbar spinal bones, which generally disintegrate first, and the femoral neck, the bone that breaks at the hip. A woman at high risk for osteoporosis should have a DEXA around the age of 40 to serve as a baseline—much like a baseline mammogram—against which to monitor future changes.

Another option is a bone density screening of the heel, which is cheaper than a DEXA (about $80, instead of the $200 to $300 often charged for a DEXA) and more readily available in some areas of the country. The machines are small and inexpensive enough that primary-

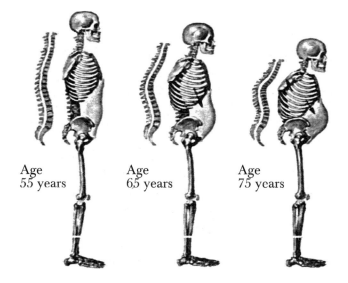

Age
55 years

Age
65 years

Age
75 years

Figure 6.2 Skeletons of women with osteoporosis.

Adapted from Netter, F.D. *The CIBA Collection of Medical Illustrations.* Summit, NJ: CIBA-Geigy Corporation: 1987: 8 (pt1): 219.

care doctors can afford to have them in their offices; if the heel scan indicates a problem, the woman can then have a DEXA for a more complete diagnosis.

Once an accurate measurement of your bone density has been obtained before menopause, a follow-up measurement can be done 12 to 18 months after your last period. If there has been a significant decrease in bone density, you are at a high personal risk for osteoporosis and should begin an aggressive preventive treatment regimen immediately. A low bone-density test for a woman in her 40s is a clear call to action.

Considering the ravages of osteoporosis, and how much it costs to treat it, you might wonder why these tests aren't done more frequently. As of July 1998, Medicare covers the cost of DEXA exams—but of course the only women who benefit from this are women 65 or older.

HMOs and health-insurance providers rarely cover the tests for younger women. Like most preventive medicine, bone scans are ultimately cost-effective. Early detection can help prevent many of the costly surgeries and physical therapy programs that individuals and the public health-care system currently pay for—not to mention the lifelong nursing-home care that half of all hip-fracture patients require.

Because women are most at risk for osteoporosis, and tests to screen for osteoporosis are rarely covered by insurance, this is another example of women's health-care concerns receiving more cavalier treatment than men's. Also, the victims of osteoporosis are largely elderly and often silent when it comes to lobbying the health-care system. But if we baby boomers live en masse into our 80s as predicted, osteoporosis may play a major role in how well we'll maintain our independence. It's in our best interest to be vocal and educate ourselves about this disease before we experience it. For more information, call or write the National Osteoporosis Foundation (listed in the Sources section at the back of this book).

Building Better Bones Now

What can you do now to prevent osteoporosis? Start by developing dense bones before you reach menopause. Calcium is essential for strong bones, and it is recommended that a menopausal woman at risk for osteoporosis take 1,500 mg daily. This is twice the normal recommended dosage and the equivalent of five 8-ounce glasses of milk a day, so unless you really like milk you'll probably need supplements to meet the requirement.

Large amounts of calcium are difficult for the body to absorb at once, so it is better to take smaller doses at regular intervals, such as 500 mg before each meal. Vitamin D helps the body absorb calcium: 500 IU of vitamin D a day is the standard recommendation, and especially vital for women who live in cloudy climates and don't get regular exposure to sunlight. Magnesium and vitamin K also aid in bone repair; vitamin K is present in many foods, including almost all vegetables, so deficiency is rare, but 600 mg of magnesium daily will round out your bone-building program.

A sedentary lifestyle sets you up for weaker bones. Both weight-bearing exercise (any activity, such as walking, where your body is forced to support its own weight) and weight-resistance exercises (such as weightlifting or working out with rubberized bands) build bone mass. It is also important to stop smoking and limit the Chardonnay and espresso, because nicotine, caffeine, and alcohol all inhibit your ability to absorb calcium.

A woman whose DEXA reveals solid bones and who has no familial predisposition toward osteoporosis may be able to prevent the disease through vitamin therapy, proper diet, exercise, and a health-conscious lifestyle. But if your DEXA indicates lighter-than-average bones, you'll need estrogen—or a bone-building drug like Fosamax.

Fosamax (alendronate) is an alternative for the prevention and treatment of osteoporosis for women who opt not to take estrogen. Fosamax stimulates bone-building activity and reduces fracture risk by 50 percent by increasing bone density at the spine and hip. It can be tough to take, however. To avoid irritating the esophagus, Fosamax should be taken on an empty stomach with an 8-ounce glass of water. You must then remain upright for 30 minutes afterward, without eating or drinking. Some women take it first thing in the morning and then shower and dress, allowing enough time to pass before they sit down to breakfast. The usual dose for the prevention of osteoporosis is 5 mg per day; 10 mg per day is needed to treat existing osteoporosis.

HRT is a powerful weapon in the battle to maintain stronger bones because estrogen not only retards bone loss but in some cases actually seems to reverse osteo-porosis by increasing bone density. This is not a quick-fix solution, however. When a woman stops HRT she will begin once again to lose bone mass at her previous rate, so a woman whose main goal in HRT is to prevent osteo-porosis will have to continue the therapy even after her menopausal symptoms subside. Recent studies have shown that taking estrogen and Fosamax together helps build bone mass at the hip, a notoriously difficult area to rehabilitate once the bone has thinned.

We spoke with one very active woman in her 40s who broke an ankle in a volleyball game. Her doctor hesitated to use pins to set the fracture because the bones surrounding the break were so brittle he feared that inserting the pin would crack them. A follow-up DEXA revealed that her bones were much lighter than average, so she began a vig-orous program of osteoporosis prevention. Her sister, who, it turned out, had the same condition, did the same. Most women are not privy to information about their bones until it is far too late for preventive medicine, which is why a screening heel scan can be helpful diagnostic tools if you suspect you may be at risk for osteoporosis.

Alzheimer's Disease

The problem: Alzheimer's disease is a degenerative disor-der of the brain, resulting over time in memory loss, behavior and personality changes, and a decline in cogni-tive abilities. This decline in brain function usually lands the person in a long-term chronic-care facility and ulti-mately leads to death.

If you've ever known a person with Alzheimer's you know that the clinical definition fails to capture the heart-break of this disease.

Forty percent of persons over age 80—almost 4 million people in the United States alone—suffer from Alzheimer's disease. This is especially alarming because the elderly are the fastest growing segment of the population. Unlike the heart or bones, which can grow strong again with medication or lifestyle changes, once the brain begins to degenerate, the process is almost impossible to reverse.

Who is at risk for Alzheimer's? You won't find a risk evaluation box in this section as you did for heart disease and osteoporosis precisely because it is hard to predict who will develop Alzheimer's. Fortunately, the Women's Health Initiative is looking at risk factors for Alzheimer's as well as heart disease, cancer, and osteoporosis; that study's findings will be out long before we baby boomers reach the Alzheimer's age bracket.

Alzheimer's seems to run in families. If your parents or grandparents suffered from it, you may be at elevated risk. But because Alzheimer's often doesn't show up until people reach their 80s, your grandparents may not have lived long enough to develop it, and your parents may not yet be at that age, leaving you unsure of your degree of genetic risk.

Women develop Alzheimer's four times more than men, perhaps because the testosterone men produce throughout life is converted into small amounts of estrogen to help to maintain brain function, and perhaps because women simply live longer. One other intriguing theory is that women who undergo dramatic drops in their estrogen levels at menopause may be at extra risk for Alzheimer's because each severe hot flash kills brain cells. (Just one more thing to worry about while you're in the office wash room sponging off after a big one!) The intensity of hot flashes has been correlated with changes in cognitive function.

The solution: What estrogen taketh away, estrogen can giveth back. Women who take HRT report that their ability to remember things improves almost immediately, but, more importantly, estrogen reduces a woman's risk of developing Alzheimer's by 40 percent. (Clinical studies show the risk being reduced by anywhere from one-third to one-half.) This may be attributed to estrogen's effect on the growth of nerve cells, improved blood flow to the brain, or due to estrogen's effect on neurotransmitters such as serotonin. Whatever the reason, if the study numbers continue to hold up, some experts believe that the prevention of Alzheimer's may become the primary reason doctors prescribe HRT and women take it.

The connection between estrogen and lower rates of Alzheimer's was first noticed in observational studies at retirement communities, most notably at one called Leisure World. Not only did fewer women on HRT develop Alzheimer's but—even more amazing considering the fact that the brain rarely regenerates—giving estrogen to women who already had Alzheimer's improved their cognitive performance. Nonsteroid anti-inflammatory drugs such as ibuprofen, taken daily in a low dose, have also been associated with a reduced risk of Alzheimer's.

Breast Cancer

The problem: HRT has been linked to a higher incidence of breast cancer, though the studies are either inconclusive or conflicting.

No other disease frightens women as much as breast cancer. Although osteoporosis and heart disease ultimately kill six times more women than cancer does, most of those women are over the age of 60. Breast cancer is scary precisely because it can strike when a woman is young and seemingly healthy: One-third of the women who die from breast cancer are under 50, meaning you may well know a woman your age who has been diagnosed with the disease. Breast cancer looms large in the minds of many perimenopausal women as something that could happen to them, so they approach estrogen therapy with suspicion.

Colon Cancer

Estrogen also cuts your risk of colon cancer, the third leading cause of cancer death in women. This particular kind of cancer is more common in women than men, and your risk begins to climb at age 40, peaking at 60 to 75.

Estrogen reduces a woman's risk for colon cancer by 40 percent; taken with aspirin, estrogen is especially effective in reducing the occurrence of the polyps that may lead to colon cancer. It is also important to eat plenty of fruits and vegetables and to keep your fiber intake high.

The American Cancer Society recommends a digital rectal exam and fecal occult blood test every year, and a flexible sigmoidoscopy every five years after the age of 50. A colonoscopy may be recommended if you have ever had a positive occult blood test or have a strong family history of colon cancer.

A link between breast cancer and HRT makes sense in theory. Women who start their periods earlier than normal or who go through a later-than-typical menopause have a higher risk of breast cancer, presumably because their bodies have been exposed to estrogen longer. Also some breast tumors grow in response to estrogen, and many women who have breast cancer respond favorably to the estrogen-blocking medication tamoxifen.

These commonsense observations have been enough to prompt concern about the connection between estrogen and breast cancer, but the trouble is that three major studies have yielded three somewhat different results. Let's start with the depressing and indisputable fact that the average American woman has a 10 percent chance of contracting breast cancer in her lifetime, and then ask: If she takes HRT, what happens to the 10 percent risk?

1. The Centers for Disease Control (CDC) concluded that if a woman has been on HRT for 15 years, her breast cancer risk rises 30 percent. (Note: A 30 percent increase in a 10 percent base risk would raise a woman's personal chances of getting breast cancer to 13 percent, not 40 percent.) Women who were on estrogen for five years or less showed no increased risk.

2. A Vanderbilt University study found no increased risk among women taking estrogen in the standard 0.625 mg dose. Because many of the subjects of the CDC study had been on estrogen for 15 years or longer, most began taking HRT in the high-dosage days of the 1970s, so some doctors argue that the Vanderbilt study is more relevant for women just beginning HRT.

3. Finally, the ongoing Nurses' Health Study conducted at Harvard University has concluded that a woman who once took estrogen but stopped has no increased breast cancer risk and that only women who have been on estrogen for more than 10 years bear the additional 30 percent risk noted in the CDC study. This means that once you stop taking estrogen, your risk drops to its initial lower level. This is curious because most carcinogens' effects (such as that of tobacco) linger in the body, raising some doubt as to whether estrogen is carcinogenic at all. The study also suggests that estrogen promotes the growth of existing tumors rather than causing new tumors to develop; that is, estrogen doesn't cause cancer, but it accelerates the growth of preexisting cancer cells.

   Because of the length of time the women were monitored and the large number of women (more than 100,000) included, the Nurses' Health Study is considered the most important breast cancer study today. The Women's Health Initiative Study, due out in 2007, will be even more conclusive, and should clear up some of the confusion about the connection between estrogen and breast cancer.

What all three studies conclude in common is that short-term use of HRT doesn't significantly increase your risk of breast cancer; a woman has to be on estrogen for more than five years before her risk is elevated. Because dosage also seems to affect breast cancer risk, some doctors advocate a 0.625 mg dose (or equivalent) of estrogen while

The Women's Health Initiative

This monumental research project, funded by the U.S. Congress with preliminary results due in 2007, focuses on women's health issues during the menopausal years. A staggering 165,000 women ages 50 to 79, the largest group ever studied, will engage in the clinical trial, which will evaluate the benefits and risks of lowfat diets, hormone replacement therapy, and calcium and vitamin D supplementation.

The accompanying observational study will monitor women of all races and backgrounds over a period of nine years to try to improve risk prediction for heart disease, breast cancer, and osteoporosis. This information will help physicians work more effectively with midlife women in the future and will be very meaningful to baby boomers as they age. Because of the sheer size and scope of the study, the Women's Health Initiative will undoubtedly lay to rest some of the uncertainty or conflicting data about the effects of HRT on women's long-term health.

Risk Factors for Breast Cancer

1. Did you begin having periods earlier than average (before the age of 12)?

2. Did you have a later-than-average menopause (after the age of 54)?

3. Were you over 30 when your first child was born? Or, are you childless?

4. Are you obese?

5. Do you have a mother or sister who contracted breast cancer before the age of 50?

6. Are you Caucasian? (Caucasian women living in the Western Hemisphere have the highest statistical rate of breast cancer in the world.)

7. Do you drink more than two alcoholic beverages a day?

the woman is going through menopause, followed by a smaller 0.3 mg dosage once she is past the age of 60 and requires less estrogen to suppress her symptoms.

Although women with personal risk factors working against them are considered to be at elevated risk, the disturbing truth is that it's extremely hard to predict who will get breast cancer. Eighty percent of the women diagnosed with the disease have no increased risk factors at all. Questions about estrogen use keep resurfacing partly because we are still years away from understanding who is most likely to get breast cancer.

Advice for Women with Family Histories of Breast Cancer

The Nurses' Health Study raises troubling issues for women with family histories of breast cancer or who have had the disease themselves. Because estrogen may accelerate the growth of existing tumors, is hormone therapy ever advisable for women at high risk for breast cancer?

Most doctors feel that it's safe to take estrogen on a short-term basis even if you have a family history of breast cancer. Many doctors say they would not hesitate to prescribe transitional HRT for a couple of years to a woman who was experiencing disruptive symptoms.

But whether or not a woman with high risk for breast cancer should take long-term HRT is a stickier question. A woman who has a mother or sister who was diagnosed with breast cancer before the age of 50 has a 25 percent chance of developing the disease; her risk rises by 30 percent with long-term HRT, putting her personal risk in the 31 to 33 percent range—frighteningly high. But does her risk really rise by a full 30 percent? No one knows. The lone study done specifically on women who have family histories of breast cancer showed that their risk rose only slightly, remaining around 25 percent, with or without HRT. But because only one study has been carried out and it used a relatively small number of subjects, HRT for these women remains a tough call to make. Results of the Women's Health Initiative should provide some answers.

In the meantime, the tiebreaker is how badly you need the therapy. If your risk for heart disease or osteoporosis equals or exceeds your risk for breast cancer, long-term HRT may still be your best choice.

Advice for Women with Personal Histories of Breast Cancer

Most doctors are reluctant to prescribe HRT for women who have had breast cancer, but even this rule is open to debate. One recent study showed that short-term use of HRT caused no cases of tumor reactivation, but that long-term use is more questionable.

Alcohol and Breast Cancer

Some of the most alarming news that has come out recently involves the link between even moderate alcohol consumption and breast cancer. Is your evening glass of wine really that dangerous?

Here are the facts. Alcohol increases the concentration of estrogen in the blood of postmenopausal women on HRT, and this elevation may be enough to promote breast cancer. In fact daily consumption of alcohol increases your chance of getting breast cancer more than HRT does. Women who drink more than 30 grams of alcohol a day—which translates to three or more glasses of wine, three or more beers, or more than two shots of liquor—have a 41 percent higher chance of developing invasive breast cancer than nondrinkers.

Fewer drinks mean less risk. A woman who has one drink a day doesn't increase her risk of cancer as much as a heavy drinker—although it does increase some. It's important to remember the math here too. Alcohol doesn't give you a 41 percent chance of developing breast cancer, but rather raises, for example, a 2 percent chance to 3 percent.

To further complicate matters, red wine, which contains antioxidants, may actually inhibit tumor growth. Until more conclusive studies are released, however, the safest course for a woman on HRT is to not drink at all or to limit herself to an occasional glass of wine.

This decision should be addressed on a case-by-case basis. Your physician should consider these factors:

1. How long has the woman been cancer-free? Many doctors offer HRT to women who have had no cancer for five years or longer, arguing that there is no evidence that estrogen aggravates successfully treated

cancer. Other doctors contend that there's no evidence that it doesn't aggravate dormant cancer and that it would be foolish to take even the slightest chance—especially considering that women who have had breast cancer bear a risk more than six times greater than normal of redeveloping the disease.

2. How badly is the patient suffering? Short-term HRT for a patient with debilitating symptoms may be recommended. Also, if a woman is already in the final stages of cancer and is suffering from severe estrogen-deficiency symptoms, her physician may prescribe HRT in an effort to improve the quality of the months or years she has left.

3. What is the patient's risk for heart disease and osteoporosis? Long-term use for a patient with no particular risk would probably not be recommended.

Tamoxifen

A drug that blocks the effects of estrogen, tamoxifen is frequently prescribed for women with breast cancer because it prevents the growth of malignant cells. Strangely enough, this anti-estrogen drug acts like estrogen in some parts of the body, offering some protection against osteoporosis and heart disease.

Tamoxifen doesn't help hot flashes, vaginal dryness, and the other transitional symptoms of perimenopause, and 5 percent of the women who take it report side effects such as nausea or bloating. But for a woman who has had breast cancer, a drug that opposes malignant cells while protecting her bones and heart can seem like a godsend. A new SERM on the market, raloxifene, may eventually turn out to be an even better option, because it seems to have no ill effects on the uterus.

Some doctors will prescribe HRT for former cancer patients if they have a particularly high risk of
heart disease or are already showing signs of rapid
bone loss.

Cancer Screening

The monthly self-exam is your first line of defense against
breast cancer. Designate a certain time each month to do
the exam—after your period, if you're still having them,
or when you pay the electric bill if you're not. If you have
any doubts about the effectiveness of your technique, ask
your doctor or nurse to show you how. An annual check by
a medical professional is an added safety net.

We all know the importance of having mammograms,
but there are several schools of thought on how often we
should have them. The American Cancer Society recommends a baseline mammogram by age 35 or before beginning HRT; after that, some physicians recommend annual
mammograms while others say that every two years will
suffice. Talk to your doctor. Your personal risk factors may
make the difference as to how often he or she advises a
mammogram.

A final note: Some women report that their doctors
started them on HRT with no discussion of breast cancer
at all. If your doctor prescribes hormone therapy without
discussing your personal breast-cancer risk and screening
techniques, that's a flashing neon sign that this person is
not equipped to help you manage your perimenopause.

The Bottom Line

One of the reasons that we're all so frightened about HRT
is that we've talked ourselves into believing that any decision we make is irreversible. It's as if we're standing at a

fork in the road with breast cancer lurking in one direction and a heart attack waiting in the other.

It's key to remember that the risk of cancer for ever-users and never-users of HRT is identical. Short-term use of HRT appears to have no effect on a woman's chances of contracting cancer, so if you need estrogen to ease you through the transitions of perimenopause, there's no reason not to take it. HRT is not a once-in-a-lifetime decision, but rather a year-by-year decision that can be altered any time. You may start on HRT, have a scary mammogram, and decide it's not worth it. You may vow, "No pills for me," then learn from a DEXA that you're losing bone mass rapidly and be forced to reconsider.

The bottom line is that you must assess your personal risk for the four big diseases discussed in this chapter, as well as your discomfort level from perimenopausal symptoms, before you make your decision about HRT (see Figure 6.3). Then reassess with each new mammogram,

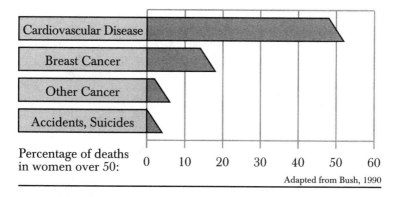

Figure 6.3 Cardiovascular Disease (CVD), including heart disease and stroke, is responsible for more than 50 percent of all deaths from specific conditions among U.S. women over age 50.

DEXA, or cholesterol test, each new symptom, and each new study. Medicine can be introduced or removed from your system as circumstances dictate.

No decision is irreversible. Estrogen does not linger in the body for years. If it did, we wouldn't go through menopause in the first place.

7

Wellness: Weight Control, Diet, and Exercise

If you just set people in motion, they'll heal themselves.
—Gabrielle Roth

Health is more than the absence of disease. Ideally, we strive for wellness—a sense of feeling energetic, alert, and in charge of our bodies and our lives. If you think of your health care as merely solving problems as they develop, you're taking a reactive approach. Wellness requires "pro-action"—heading off pain and disease before they occur and focusing not just on the isolated symptom, but on the bigger issues of energy, relaxation, balance, and nutrition.

If you've thought about making changes—exercising more, eating better, giving up coffee, alcohol, or cigarettes—perimenopause is the perfect time to act on those good intentions. A short-term problem, such as insomnia or a sudden weight gain, may initially prompt you, but the changes you make now will help determine not only how long you live, but how well you live.

Weight Control

Are we doomed to gain weight during the menopausal years? Most women do, and those who are already obese gain more than women who enter menopause at a normal weight. Women on average gain 10 to 15 pounds after menopause; obese women gain an average of 21 to 23 pounds.

In many cases, the weight gain can be traced to a lower metabolic rate. During perimenopause, your lean body mass begins to decrease and your fat body mass begins to increase. Fat is inert, and your body doesn't have to work very hard to sustain it. So the fatter you become, the less fuel your body requires. Do we sense a cycle beginning here? Because a stalled metabolism means you're burning fewer calories, you can gain weight even if you're eating the same amount you've eaten for years.

This is precisely why midlife weight gains frustrate so many women. They argue that they aren't overeating—and if you define overeating as eating more than you used to, they aren't. But if an inactive lifestyle and lack of muscle mass have combined to slow your metabolic rate, you can gain weight on 1,800 calories a day—which hardly anyone in our culture would consider overeating. By taking in only 200 more calories a day than you expend, you will gain approximately 20 pounds in a year.

Do Hormones Affect Weight Gain?

Hormone replacement therapy doesn't seem to impact perimenopausal weight gain. A recent study of women who opted for HRT and those who didn't showed similar weight gains in the hormone-treated women and the control group. However, hormones may affect where you carry the weight.

The fat cells postmenopausal women accumulate tend to cluster around their abdomen in the "apple" distribution associated more with men, that is, the classic "beer belly." Prior to menopause, most women who are overweight have a "pear" body type, with their fat sitting mainly on their hips and thighs. Because women tend to start out pear-shaped and become more apple-shaped after menopause, it makes sense that this new fat distribution may be due to hormonal changes.

Studies are inconclusive, but have suggested that HRT reverses the menopausal tendency toward apple-shaped fat distribution, and that it encourages future fat to stay in the pear-shaped distribution. This is not merely a cosmetic debate: Fat in the abdominal area is far more dangerous to the heart than fat in the hip and thigh area.

How Fat Is Fat?

DEXA, the same test that measures bone density, can also be used to measure body fat percentages. A new type of scale, which can measure body fat instead of weight, is available in some clinics as well. A submersion test, based on the fact that fat floats and lean body mass sinks, is another accurate way of calculating how much fat you're carrying. If you can't travel to a hospital or full-service spa for one of these tests, at least ask your doctor or a trainer at the local gym for a caliper skin test. A device that measures the amount of surface fat by lightly pinching the skin on the arm and hip, calipers can give you a basic idea of where you stand.

Your body-fat percentage is vital information, for a scale only tells half of the story. Weight doesn't affect our long-term health as much as our body fat percentage. Some thin-looking but sedentary women have more fat than the desirable 20 to 25 percent range, and, conversely, some active women weigh more than you would guess. This was dramatically proven to us when an aerobics instructor, whose body every woman in the class admired, climbed on the spa scales to prove she weighed 145 pounds. Anyone would have guessed she was 20 pounds lighter, but this was a woman with very toned muscles—and muscle weighs more than fat but takes up less room. At 145 pounds she had an enviably low body fat measurement of 18 percent.

Muscle Mass: The Missing Component in Weight Loss

The vast majority of us are not professional athletes, nor do we necessarily aspire to have vein-bulging muscles. But any woman can increase her muscle mass and raise her metabolism. Obviously, exercise burns fat while you are exercising, but by forcing the body to work harder to maintain its newer, hungrier muscles, exercise also helps you burn more fat even while resting.

Adults on average lose a half-pound of muscle mass every year after age 20; in women over 35, the rate of loss accelerates to one pound a year. With each lost pound of muscle, you burn 50 fewer calories a day. Happily, the formula also works in reverse. With each pound of muscle you develop, your body will require 50 additional calories a day. This means that if an active 130-pound woman has just five more pounds of muscle than an inactive 130-pound woman, the active woman can eat 250 calories a day more than the inactive woman. If the inactive woman took in the same number of calories as the active woman she would gain more than 20 pounds in a single year.

For this reason, an increased activity level is more vital than diet to the menopausal woman who is fighting obesity. If your food intake hasn't increased, but your weight has, don't try eating less. Try moving more.

Exercise

The advantages to regular physical activity are numerous and well documented. Exercise:

- maintains bone density, especially if you do weight-bearing and weight-resistance exercises
- maintains muscle mass
- increases metabolism, burning calories and fat
- reduces the risks of cancer, diabetes, and heart disease
- reduces stress
- alleviates many of the symptoms of menopause (including some you might not guess, such as hot flashes)
- helps former smokers stay off the cigarettes
- may boost the immune system, making you less vulnerable to communicable diseases such as colds and flu
- helps maintain flexibility and joint movement as you age

Types of Exercise

The three basic types of exercise are aerobics, weight resistance, and flexibility training.

Aerobic Exercise   Aerobic activities include walking, running, swimming, biking, and most group fitness classes such as step or low-impact aerobics. The primary function of aerobics is to burn fat and work the heart and lungs. If the aerobics are weight bearing (activities such as walking or bench stepping, where the body is upright and supports its own weight), aerobic activity also increases bone density and muscle strength.

Note: For women with arthritis or a history of joint injuries, swimming is an excellent cardiovascular workout, and water aerobics are also a good option, because a well-choreographed class will not only challenge you aerobically but also provide some resistance and flexibility work.

Aerobic activity for 30 minutes three times a week will protect the heart, but if your main goal is weight loss, you'll have to do far more than that. To burn fat, you'll need to exercise in your target rate zone for 45 to 60 minutes, five to six days a week.

Weight Resistance   Weight training doesn't have to mean an hour on the Nautilus machines, although you might enjoy this more than you would guess. You can maintain muscle mass with handheld weights or special rubber bands that create resistance. To work the abdominal muscles and strengthen the torso, crunches should be part of your exercise routine.

Some women skip this important step in fitness, arguing that they don't want a muscle-bound look. In truth, very few women have enough testosterone in their systems to produce huge muscles, but all women past 40 need to do some sort of weight-resistance training for four key reasons:

- It slows the loss of bone mass and helps you avoid osteoporosis.
- It helps you maintain muscle mass, especially in the upper body, which is often ignored even by women who do aerobic exercise on a regular basis.
- Because it requires more energy to sustain muscle than fat, a woman with a high percentage of muscle mass will be able to eat more calories without gaining weight than a woman with a low percentage of muscle mass.

♦ Strength is empowering. The very nature of weight training makes it easy to see incremental progress; if you were doing 40 pounds on the bicep machine at the YMCA last week and are doing 50 this week, that's a definitive change. Some women find it easier to maintain their motivation with weight training than with any other type of exercise.

If you want to build muscle mass, not just maintain it, join a gym and consider a few sessions with a personal trainer. Most large gyms have trainers on staff and you can often hire them for three or four sessions, a worthwhile investment if you've never lifted weights. A trainer will make sure that your form is correct, which dramatically lowers your chance of injury, and will also help you determine the best weight to begin with for the various machines. Once your program is underway, it's not a bad idea to schedule a single session every three months or so, especially when you feel it's time to increase your weights or repetitions.

In general, you should weight train for at least an hour a week. This could be divided into two 30-minute sessions, or three 20-minute sessions. (An hourly session once a week is less effective, but still better than nothing.) Work the biggest muscles—legs, back, and chest—first, before moving onto smaller muscle groups in the shoulders or arms. If you're working at an appropriate weight level, you should be able to do 10 to 12 repetitions, slowly, without compromising your form. Always let at least 48 hours pass between sessions so your muscles have time to rest and repair.

Flexibility The fitness component most likely to be ignored, flexibility exercise is especially important for women as they age. Many kinds of flexibility work, such as yoga, ballet, or simple stretching, have the added bonus of reducing stress and improving sleep.

As with weight training, you should aim to do flexibility work for at least an hour a week, although it's virtually impossible to overtrain in this area and you should certainly feel free to do as much flexibility work as you enjoy. The basic 60 minutes a week can be divided up any way that suits you: 15 minutes four times a week, or 20 minutes three times a week makes sense for many women.

Five minutes of stretching after an aerobic workout is always a good idea, too, and most responsibly run classes incorporate stretching into the cool-down period. The purpose of most postaerobic stretching, however, is to avoid soreness or cramps. To actually increase your flexibility, consider signing up for a class in yoga, tai chi chuan, or dance.

There are also excellent videotapes on the market if you'd rather exercise at home. We like the *Yoga Journal* series called "Living Arts," which features a wide variety of tapes for all experience levels. If you're just starting out, "A.M. and P.M. Yoga" featuring Rodney Yee and Patricia

Target Heart Rate Zone

You can find your target heart rate range using the following formula:

1. Subtract your age from 220.
2. Multiply that number by 0.6. This is the lower end of your range.
3. Multiply the same number by 0.85. This is the higher end of your range.

In other words, during exercise, a healthy 45-year-old woman would have a target heart rate range of 105 to 148.

Walden is an easy orientation to basic stretches, conveniently presented in a 15-minute morning session and 20-minute evening session. These tapes are widely available in bookstores and video stores or you can call (800) 2-LIV-ING for the Living Arts catalog.

Exercising for Weight Loss

Make no mistake: Exercise is an essential component of any weight-loss program and study after study has shown that while dieting may take pounds off, *90 percent of the people who diet without exercising will regain the weight.* (Note the italics—we'd put it in neon lights if we could!)

Optimum fat burning occurs when you exercise at about 70 percent of your maximum heart rate, which for a 45-year-old woman would be about 125 beats a minute. How do you know that you're in your target range? There are three ways to check:

> **Pulse Check:** After you've been exercising for about 10 minutes, put two fingertips to your throat just below your jaw and find your pulse. Then, using a clock or a watch with a second hand, count your heartbeats for 6 seconds, starting with zero for the first beat. Let's say you feel 12 beats. If you add a zero to this number, you're in effect multiplying a 6-second count by 10 and estimating how many times your heart is beating in a minute. A count of 12 indicates a heart rate of about 120.

> **Perceived Exertion Method:** This is a fancy way of saying that if you feel like you're getting ready to pass out, you probably are. In your ideal training range, you should feel like you're working fairly hard—as one aerobics instructor put it, able to talk but not quite able to sing. Obviously, perceived exertion is a

subjective means of measurement, more helpful in keeping you from overtraining than in determining a precise pulse rate. If you are gasping for breath or begin to feel dizzy, ease up.

Heart Rate Monitor: Once only used for professional athletes, heart rate monitors are now widely available at sporting goods stores for about $100 to $150. In most models, an elastic band attaches across your chest to count your heartbeats and convey this information to a watch-like device that straps onto your wrist.

Many monitors come with an option that lets you program in your high and low ranges; the watch will then beep if you drop out of range, signaling that you're working too hard or not hard enough. When Kim bought a monitor she was surprised to learn how frequently she was dropping out of her training range while on her daily walk; waiting at a stoplight or becoming too absorbed in conversation with a friend, she was often slowing down her pace without being aware of it. A healthy woman's heart can recover—that is, slow down—in just a matter of seconds.

This is important information because fat burning requires you to not only *attain* your target heart range but to *maintain* that range for 45 to 60 minutes. Many women who complain they've been walking for months with no noticeable benefits probably aren't walking quite fast enough or they need to choose a hillier, more demanding route.

On the flip side, a heart rate monitor also keeps you from zooming up to 170 during a demanding step class. Even the most conscientious instructor rarely stops the class for more than one or two heart rate checks, and if you haven't been exercising regularly you could easily be working out of your target zone for at least part of a class.

Body Mass Index

The Body Mass Index (BMI) expresses the relationship between a person's weight and height. It is calculated as weight in kilograms, divided by height in meters squared. The best way to determine a good weight range for you is to use the BMI formula. Grab a calculator.

1. Multiply your present weight by 704. This is x.
2. Multiply your height in inches by your height in inches. This is y.
3. Divide x by y.
4. The result is your body mass index, which should fall somewhere between 18 and 25. To be below 18 or above 25 is to put your health at risk.

For example, let's say you are 5 feet, 4 inches (64 inches) tall and weigh 142 pounds. Multiply 142 by 704 for a total of 99,968. Next, multiply 64 by 64 for a total of 4,096. Divide 99,968 by 4,096 to result in a BMI of around 24. You're within a healthy range, although near the high end, and should be aware that if you gain 10 pounds your BMI will be in the unhealthy range.

How Does Exercise Counteract Calorie Intake?

For many women, exercising six hours a week within their target range will in and of itself be enough to help them lose weight. If you'd like to keep an exercise journal and be a bit more scientific about the process, begin with the fact that the most successful weight-loss programs are a combination of a slight reduction of calories taken in through food and a slight increase in the number of calories burned through exercise.

A pound of fat equals 3,500 calories, so if you'd like to lose a pound of fat a week—a reasonable goal—you can:

♦ eat 3,500 fewer calories;

♦ burn off 3,500 calories through exercise;

♦ or eat 2,000 fewer calories and burn off 2,000 calories through exercise.

The last option is both the easiest and the best. (You've undoubtedly noticed that it produces a 4,000-calorie deficit, which is okay because we always seem to be eating a little more and exercising a little less than we think we are.) In the next section we'll discuss how to slightly modify your food intake to encourage long-term weight loss, but for the time being, let's focus on exercise. What does it take to burn off 2,000 calories a week?

Based on a woman's weight, Table 7.1 estimates how many calories she will burn during 1 hour or 45 minutes of various types of exercise.

As you can see from the table, while the idea of burning off 2,000 calories each week through exercise may seem overwhelming, for a 150-pound woman it pretty much comes down to a 45-minute walk three times a week and a couple of 60-minute aerobics classes. A definite time commitment, but also definitely doable.

Walking

Remember when bananas were being touted as the ideal food? Actually, no one food can give you everything you need, nor can one exercise, but walking is the closest thing we have to the "banana" in the exercise world. A 30-minute walk will give you aerobic benefits with minimal expense and chance of injury; gradually increase your

	130 lbs.	140 lbs.	150 lbs.	160 lbs.	170 lbs.	180 lbs.
Aerobics class	460/ 345	500/ 375	534/ 400	567/ 425	605/ 453	638/ 478
Step aerobics class	530/ 397	576/ 432	616/ 462	654/ 490	697/ 522	736/ 552
Walking (3.5 mph) or elliptical trainer	400/ 300	434/ 325	465/ 348	493/ 369	526/ 394	555/ 416
Swimming	480/ 360	521/ 390	558/ 418	592/ 444	631/ 473	666/ 500
Cycling (10–12 mph)	410/ 307	445/ 334	476/ 357	506/ 380	539/ 404	569/ 426

Table 7.1 Calorie burn-off (calories burned in 1 hour/calories burned in 45 minutes).

duration until you're up to an hour and you'll burn a lot more fat.

Another way to increase the intensity of a walking program is to interval train. Simply put, this involves adding short, one- to three-minute periods in which you work harder, raising your heart rate to about 85 percent of your target range. You can do this by either increasing your speed or, if you're using a treadmill, increasing the incline.

An interval training session on a treadmill might go something like this: Begin with a five-minute warm-up of relatively slow walking, around 3.2 mph. Then increase your speed to 3.5 to 4 mph, or whatever pace you have determined keeps your heart rate at about 70 percent of your target range. After five minutes, either increase your speed to 4 to 4.5 mph, or raise the machine to a 5 percent incline. When you're first beginning, make these inter-vals only a minute in duration, but over the course of time, gradually increase the intervals to a length of three min-utes. After each interval, drop back to five minutes of walking at your normal pace until you have walked for a total of at least 45 minutes, then finish with a five-minute cool-down.

Intervals are a little trickier when you're walking out-doors, and must rely on variations of pace, because it's unlikely you'll encounter a hill exactly every five minutes. A heart rate monitor is a big help, because it gives you feedback on just how fast you'll have to walk to get your heart rate up to 85 percent of its target range during an interval.

Walking magazine is a great source of information on interval training and other subjects of interest to serious walkers. You can find *Walking* on the newsstands or by writ-ing to P.O. Box 5011, Harlan, IA 51593-2511.

For a walking program to have lasting benefits you'll need to forestall boredom and burnout. One way to do this is to cross-train. Women who incorporate more than one type of activity into their exercise programs—they swim three days a week and walk three, for example, or join a gym that offers a variety of classes—stay with it longer than those who grimly follow the same routine every day.

Even varying your route can fight boredom, and some women listen to books or music on headsets, which is especially good if you walk on a track or treadmill and don't have to worry about staying alert to traffic. "It's my think time," says one woman who has walked her way through the *New York Times* best-seller list, three miles at a clip. Finding an exercise partner can also hold you to it, either because you know a friend is waiting to walk with you on your lunch hour or because the gym becomes not only a place to work out, but also your social time. Seeing friends on a regular basis is good for the heart, too.

How Am I Supposed to Work This All In?

As we've already mentioned, if you're at a healthy weight and are exercising solely for health benefits you can get by with 30 minutes of aerobics three times a week. On the other three days, you can use your 30 minutes of exercise time in a combination of weight training and stretching. Or, if you'd rather not work out every day, do aerobics three times a week, with each session followed by weight training and stretching. Either way, it adds up to three or four hours a week, a small amount of time for all the pay-offs of exercise.

For weight loss, you'll need to triple that investment of time, mostly in the area of aerobics: Work aerobically for 45 to 60 minutes five to six times a week, and devote at least two hours weekly to weight resistance and flexibility work. Some women follow a schedule of a 60-minute aerobic workout five days a week, with, say, the Monday-Wednesday-Friday workouts followed by weight resistance training and the Tuesday-Thursday workouts followed by flexibility exercises. That's an hour and a half of exercise each weekday, but you get the weekends off.

Many women tell us that they intend to exercise after work, and then are either too tired or they get swept up in the 6 P.M. madness of working mothers. The busiest people often have the most success when they exercise in the morning, which is often the most manageable time of the day. It's important to find the time that best suits you and stick with it because, although you may be exercising primarily to lose weight, your health demands that you keep working out even after you reach your BMI goal. Regular exercise is a major component of fighting the diseases of middle age.

Finally, don't let the time squeeze tempt you to skip the weight training and flexibility work. Weighing 125 pounds will do you little good if you can't carry a bag of groceries, or stoop to lift them if they fall. Although the weight-loss benefits of regular exercise are undeniable, the primary focus should always be balance and health.

Some Commonsense Precautions

1. If you're over 35 and have health-risk factors or have been extremely inactive, see your doctor before starting an exercise program. If you're over 50 when you begin, you should definitely see your doctor and request an evaluation to determine your precise target heart rate.

2. Exercise must be regular. A weekend blitz—where a sedentary person suddenly leaps into six straight hours of skiing—is more dangerous than helpful.

3. Stop if you feel short of breath, a muscle strain, joint pain, or numbness and tingling, especially in the chest or arms.

4. Use the right shoes. Exercise has become shoe-specific, with walking shoes available for walking, step shoes for step aerobics, and many kinds of running and aerobic dance shoes. At $60 a pop for a good pair of workout shoes, you may be tempted to use one pair for every activity, but don't. An investment in proper shoes is far cheaper than a trip to the orthopedic surgeon.

5. Should you exercise when you feel sick? Use the "neck check" to decide. If your ailment is above the neck—a headache, stuffy nose, or sneezing—try exercising for 10 minutes and then evaluate how you feel. If you feel fine, continue. But if your complaint is below the neck—a bad chest cough, stomach pain, or muscle strain—skip a day or two.

6. Drink eight ounces of water before and after exercising. Don't rely on thirst as an indicator of how much water you need; if you're thirsty you're already water-depleted.

7. If the temperature plus humidity equals 150, exercise indoors.

8. If you need instruction, get it. Your local YMCA or community college probably sponsors aerobics classes, running classes, even tips on walking and biking. It is especially essential to receive instruction with weight training and flexibility exercises. Books or exercise tapes can give you ideas on how to get started, but if you plan to go past the basics, take a class and ask the instructor to check your technique while lifting or stretching.

9. Sports such as golf and tennis are fun and a great way to socialize, but because the nature of the sports require you to constantly start and stop your movement, they rarely keep your heart rate consistently high enough to qualify as aerobic exercise. If you want to build your stamina, maintain heart health, or lose weight, choose a continuous-movement activity such as walking, swimming, or aerobic dance classes.

10. Don't overlook the importance of regularly getting eight hours of sleep. Many women, chronically exhausted after years of getting by on five or six hours a night, swear they don't have the strength to exercise. Sleep deprivation can also short-circuit your efforts to eat sensibly, because an afternoon energy slump makes it even more tempting to reach for that Snickers bar. If you seem to have a time of day when you compulsively snack, try meditating or taking a 10-minute catnap before you eat. Perhaps you're mistaking exhaustion for hunger.

Diet

In the middle of all the debate about high-carbohydrate, lowfat diets versus the reemerging high-protein diet, don't lose sight of one simple thing: Calories count. The basis of all permanent weight loss is eating fewer calories than you expend through activity.

How Many Calories Should You Eat?

Metabolism is a highly individualized thing and two women who eat and exercise the same amount may end up with very different looking bodies, an injustice you've undoubtedly noticed. The best way to determine how many calories your body needs to function is to keep a food diary for a week. Weigh yourself, then buy a calorie counter and a spiral notebook and write down everything you eat, including the cream in your coffee and that Andes mint you ate after lunch. Be sure to include the weekend in this little experiment, because your eating patterns are apt to be very different on a Sunday than on a Wednesday.

At the end of the week, weigh yourself again. If you've chosen a typical week, your weight should be the same as when you began and you'll have a good sense of how many calories it takes to sustain your current weight at your current activity level. Let's say you find that you're maintaining your weight of 150 pounds on 2,300 calories a day, but you'd like to weigh 130. You can lose a pound a week either by eating 500 fewer calories a day or by reducing your caloric intake by 300 calories and exercising enough to burn an additional 300 calories a day. In other words, if you remain only lightly active, you can lose weight on 1,800 calories, but if you're willing to increase your activity level, you can lose the same amount of weight on 2,000 calories.

Not everyone is going to take the time to keep a weekly food diary, so another alternative is to follow this formula:

Multiply your goal weight by 11. The result will be your resting metabolic rate, the number of calories your body needs just to keep your heart beating, your food digested, and your breathing regular. Let's say you'd like to weigh 130. Your resting metabolic rate would be 1,430.

Now add in how many calories you need for activity.

♦ If you're sedentary, that is, you sit for most of the day and don't exercise on a regular basis, multiply your resting metabolic rate by 0.2.

♦ If you're lightly active, that is, you walk several blocks to lunch and work out occasionally, multiply your resting metabolic rate by 0.3.

♦ If you're moderately active, that is, you work out on a regular basis and move around a fair amount in your daily routine, multiply your resting metabolic rate by 0.4.

♦ If you're very active, that is, an athlete in training or someone who does physically active work, multiply your resting metabolic rate by 0.5.

Most women in their 40s fall into the lightly or moderately active categories. If you want to weigh 130 and you're moderately active, you'll multiply your base count of 1,430 calories by 0.4, for a total of 572. Mystery solved. In order to weigh 130, you'll need to work out on a regular basis and eat only about 2,000 calories a day. If you're only lightly active, you need to consume about 1,860 calories. (Notice how similar these figures are to the estimates based on the previously mentioned food diary method.)

If you're a veteran of the dieting wars, having struggled to hold yourself down to 1,000 calories, the idea of losing weight on 1,800 to 2,000 calories a day probably sounds absurd. But any diet of less than 1,500 calories makes it nearly impossible to meet your nutritional needs and also causes your body to "reset" its metabolism. Our bodies are naturally self-defensive, and if yours thinks it's starving, it will go on metabolic cruise control, burning fewer calories.

It gets worse. Hardly anyone can stay on a low-calorie diet for long. If you fall into a cycle of yo-yo dieting, or alternating weeks of severe caloric restriction with binges, your body will lose a combination of fat, water, and lean muscle mass during the periods of intense dieting. The loss of muscle mass will slow your metabolic rate, and, when you regain the weight—as you almost inevitably will—it will all be in the form of fat. Let's check back in on our hypothetical (or perhaps not so hypothetical) woman who is trying to go from 150 pounds to 130. If she crash diets and loses 20 pounds, and then regains them, she'll be back to the same weight she started from, but her body fat percentage will be higher, and her metabolic rate lower.

But the worst news of all is that severe caloric restriction affects your brain function. A woman in perimenopause, already subject to mood swings and concentration lapses, will only make things tougher on herself if she tries to cut her caloric intake to below 1,500 calories a day.

High Protein vs. High Carbohydrates: What to Believe?

For years the lowfat, low-protein, high-carbohydrate diet reigned supreme. Then a new wave of diet books, arguing that Americans were getting pudgier than ever on all these fat-free snacks, began advising a return to the high-protein diet. Because you probably know people who have lost—and regained—weight on both diets, it can be very confusing.

The high-carbohydrate diet is certainly more in line with government recommendations for a healthy diet and the classic food pyramid. But it's also true that fat and protein increase your feelings of satiety—that is, if you've had a scrambled egg and piece of bacon for breakfast you not only feel fuller than you would with a breakfast of cereal or toast, but you also maintain that fuller feeling throughout the morning. People who report that their energy levels go up and down on a high-carbohydrate diet often find that they can avoid the energy crashes by adding more protein and fat to their diets.

Many of the high-protein books go beyond this commonsense approach, however, advising that you not only add more protein but that you make protein your primary food, drastically restricting your intake of carbohydrates. This flies in the face of governmental recommendations that as a nation we need to increase our intake of foods high in antioxidants and fiber, especially fruits and vegetables.

A problem that both approaches share is that it becomes extremely boring to eat one kind of food all the time, setting you up to crave the forbidden fruits—or pasta. Most of our meals, and certainly most restaurant meals, are a mixture of fat, protein, and carbohydrates, and following these diets often proves so difficult over time that people throw in the towel, even if they've lost some weight.

The solution? A diet low in fat and high in complex carbohydrates is still your best bet from a health perspective, but you can make this regimen easier to follow if you have some protein at every meal. At the height of the high-carb craze, protein was treated as one of the bad guys, but in truth it is essential for energy, especially if you're weight training and making an effort to increase your muscle mass. (Kim's personal trainer urged her to eat a bit of protein each morning before going to her weight-training session and it made a huge difference.)

The high-protein camp has another good idea when they advise us to eat five small meals a day instead of three larger ones. Healthy midmorning and afternoon snacks—fruit, half a turkey sandwich, or crackers and cheese—can keep your hunger under control, and studies have shown that as we age, we lose our ability to easily digest and metabolize huge meals.

The bottom line: You may need to be eating more protein than you are now, or at least spreading your protein intake more evenly throughout the entire day. Carbohydrates are still the key to a nutritionally balanced diet, but be conscious of the calorie count. Many "healthy" foods like pasta and bread are calorie-dense, and if you eat too much of them, you'll gain weight. And excess body fat from overindulging in whole-grain lasagna is just as dangerous as body fat from eating too many Oreos. If you've read the previous section, you have a good idea of how many calories you need to maintain a healthy weight; the idea is to eat a wide variety of foods from each category without exceeding your personal limit.

Understanding the Dietary Pyramid

Let's work our way down the pyramid shown in Figures 7.1a and 7.1b. Americans tend to undereat the foods that form the bottom of the pyramid—fruits, vegetables, and complex carbohydrates such as bread, pasta, cereal, and rice. A recent study indicated that the average American eats one vegetable a day.

Further up the pyramid, fats, dairy foods, nuts, and animal proteins are calorie-dense because of their high fat content. One gram of fat has nine calories, so with these foods you take in lots of calories, even through a small amount of food. Pure fats—oils, butter, mayonnaise, and salad dressings—are obvious trouble for people trying to watch their weight, but, unless defatted, dairy products are also apt to derive most of their caloric content from fat, not protein.

Protein has four calories per gram, so pure protein is not terribly dense in calories. Unfortunately, our protein rarely comes to us straight. Beef is marbleized with fat, chicken is served with the skin left on, fish is deep-fried. Lean proteins such as fish, shellfish, skinless chicken, and red meat that has been trimmed of fat are fine.

One gram of carbohydrate also has four calories, meaning you can eat a lot of food and still lose weight if you choose from the bottom of pyramid. But Americans have trouble figuring what constitutes "a lot." It's safe to say that what you consider a serving size and what the dieticians who create the food charts consider a serving size are not the same thing. Remember, these are the people who claim you can feed a family of eight on one box of spaghetti.

Portion Size

If you look at the grains section of the food pyramid, a serving size is 1 slice of bread, ½ cup cooked rice or pasta, or 1 ounce of cereal. When you pour a bowl of cereal, you're more likely eating 3 ounces, and ½ cup of pasta fills a saucer, not a plate. So while eight servings of grains may seem like an impossible goal, it actually translates into a bowl of cereal for breakfast, a sandwich at lunch, and spaghetti for dinner.

Take the time to measure out 4 ounces of meat or 1.5 ounces of cheese, and to pour ½ cup of rice onto a plate. To help you visualize, 4 ounces of meat is about the same size as a deck of cards, and the average amount of meat recommended for women is 5 to 6 ounces a day. Many women who struggle with midlife weight gain aren't eating enormous amounts of food or necessarily making unhealthy dietary choices, but they are often clueless as to what constitutes portion size, especially if they eat out often. Spend a week—perhaps the week you're monitoring

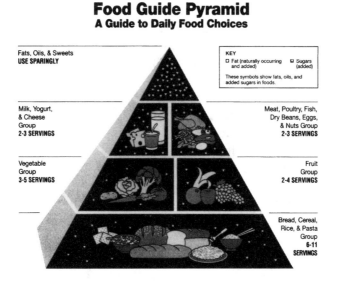

Figure 7.1a Food Pyramid.

your typical food intake as recommended earlier—weighing and measuring everything you eat. Sure, it's tedious, but it will help you more accurately "eyeball" portion sizes later, and the ability to correctly estimate portion size and the approximate calorie count of food is a huge weapon in your battle against midlife weight gain.

Restaurant Eating

If you think you're confused about proper portion size, consider the chef at the local bistro. Working women find themselves eating out frequently, and restaurant portions are huge, with evening meals sometimes topping out at 2,000 calories. Unless you're a lumberjack by trade, this spells trouble.

How to Use the Daily Food Guide

What counts as one serving?

Bread, Cereal, Rice, and Pasta
1 slice of bread
½ cup of cooked rice or pasta
½ cup of cooked cereal
1 ounce of ready-to-eat cereal

Vegetables
½ cup of chopped raw or cooked vegetables
1 cup of leafy raw vegetables

Fruit
1 whole fruit or melon wedge
¾ cup of juice
½ cup of canned fruit
¼ cup of dried fruit

Milk, Yogurt, and Cheese
1 cup of milk or yogurt
1½ to 2 ounces of cheese

Meat, Poultry, Fish, Dry Beans, Eggs, and Nuts
2½ to 3 ounces of cooked lean meat, poultry, or fish
Count ½ cup of cooked beans or 1 egg or 2 tablespoons of peanut butter as 1 ounce of lean meat (about ⅓ serving).

Fats, Oils, and Sweets
LIMIT CALORIES FROM THESE, especially if you need to lose weight.

How many servings do you need each day?

	Women & some older adults	Children, teen girls active women & most men	Teen boys & active men
Calorie level*	about 1,600	about 2,200	about 2,800
Bread group	6	9	11
Vegetable group	3	4	5
Fruit group	2	3	4
Milk group**	2–3	2–3	2–3
Meat group	2, for a total of 5 ounces	2, for a total of 6 ounces	3, for a total of 7 ounces

*These are the calorie levels if you choose lowfat, lean foods from the 5 major food groups and use foods from the fats, oils, and sweets groups sparingly.
**Women who are pregnant or breast-feeding, teenagers, and young adults to age 24 need 3 servings.

Figure 7.1b How to interpret the food pyramid.

Three solutions:

- Rather than eating fast food for lunch, brown bag it. If you must eat out at lunch, don't assume a salad is automatically your best choice. Considering the fat and calorie count of most toppings and dressings, you're likely better off with a sandwich, especially if you leave off the mayo. Soups are another good choice, a long as you steer clear of the cream-based varieties.

- When the waiter plunks down a platter of food in front of you, ask for a doggie bag immediately and wrap up half the meal. Or split an entree with a friend. The $1 sharing fee some restaurants tack on for extra plates is a real bargain when you consider the price of liposuction.

- If you're on the road and doggie bags aren't a practical solution, order a salad or soup with an appetizer instead of an entree.

Three Excellent Resources

Three of the best books we've found on the subjects of diet and exercise are *Self's Better Body Book* by the editors of *Self* magazine (Condé Nast Books, $24.95), *Strong Women Stay Young* by Dr. Miriam Nelson (Bantam, $12.95), and the *Complete Idiot's Guide to Losing Weight* by Susan McQuillan and Edward Saltzman (Alpha Books, $17.95). The *Self's* guide gives excellent advice on all types of exercise, and *Strong Women Stay Young* is an informative introduction to weight training for all ages. Although buying it may make you feel like you're announcing to the world that you're both fat *and* stupid, the *Idiot's Guide* is actually a compilation of the best weight loss advice from dozens of different sources.

Make Changes Gradually . . . and Permanently

Don't try to make all the changes at once. Gradually work healthy eating into your lifestyle and increase exercise time and intensity, so that you'll stick with it. Dramatic pledges such as, "I'll hold to 10 fat grams a day," or, "I'll never eat fast food again!" lead to dramatic lapses. Try instead to look at these as permanent changes: eating less fat instead of no fat, going out for two lunches a week and brown-bagging the rest, choosing the Ben and Jerry's Cherry Garcia frozen yogurt over the Cherry Garcia ice cream. This food plan is designed to help you feel better, not punish you for all past sins.

Even with such realistic goals, you may still hit the dreaded plateaus, but if you're holding to your food plan without continuing to lose weight, don't give in to the temptation to cut your calorie intake drastically. A far better response is to increase your exercise time, perhaps walking both in the morning and the evening, while keeping your food intake steady.

8

❦

Nutrition, Detoxification, and Stress Relief

It's easier to stay well than to get well.
—Sign in a Michigan gift shop

Nutrition sounds complicated, but there are three basic rules that, if followed, will go a long way toward cutting your risk of disease:

1. Increase the level of antioxidants and phytochemicals in your body by eating more fruits and vegetables.
2. Cut back on fat.
3. Increase your fiber intake.

Let's look at each in more detail.

Step 1: Increase Your Antioxidants

The antioxidants vitamins A, C, and E have been linked to decreased risks of cancer and heart disease. The body burns fuel through oxidation, and toxic substances called free radicals are released. Antioxidants pick up the free radicals before they can enter the organs and help the body excrete them.

Antioxidants have gotten tremendous amounts of press recently, and there is even some speculation that they are especially beneficial for people who live in an urban environment or are exposed to pollution. But while we wait for studies to conclude just how much good these antioxidants can do, it's beyond dispute that they do good, and that the American diet is woefully deficient in the foods that contain them: green or yellow vegetables, citrus fruits, and wheat.

As you can see from Table 8.1, the Alliance for Aging Research recommends daily amounts of antioxidants that are up to four times higher than the current recommended daily allowance (RDA) from the FDA.

Unless you are already taking vitamin supplements or are unusually health-conscious, you're probably falling short of even the minimum requirements. It's often said that adults should receive all the recommended daily amounts of vitamins and minerals through a healthy diet, but probably no more than 25 percent do. You know yourself. If you're more apt to hit the drive-through than pack a salad for lunch, face the facts and start taking vitamin and mineral supplements. Aim for dosages between the higher and lower recommendations. Anything the body doesn't need, it will excrete, leading to rather expensive

	FDA	Alliance for Aging Research
Vitamin A	10 mg	30 mg
Vitamin C	250 mg	1,000 mg
Vitamin E	100 IU	400 IU

Table 8.1 Antioxidant RDA.

urine—but better that than courting a health problem that you could avoid through such a simple preventive measure as taking a multivitamin.

In the sections that follow, we'll discuss the daily requirements of various vitamins and minerals, and the foods that are rich in them.

Vitamin A/Beta-Carotene

This antioxidant is primarily found in green, leafy vegetables, yellow vegetables, and yellow fruits: carrots, spinach, squash, broccoli, lettuce, peaches, apricots, and sweet potatoes.

Your daily beta-carotene needs can be met with 2 to 3 cups of these vegetables or fruits, or with a 30 mg supplement.

Vitamin C

Opinions as to the optimal daily quantity of this antioxidant range from 250 to 1,000 mg. Vitamin C is found in tomatoes, citrus fruits (oranges, grapefruits, tangerines, lemons, limes), broccoli, red and yellow peppers, celery, cauliflower, kiwi fruit, and cantaloupe.

If you're not consuming two fruits or glasses of juice a day plus at least one vegetable from the list, consider taking a 500 mg supplement.

Vitamin E

This antioxidant has the added benefit of eliminating bad cholesterol (LDL). It is found in bran, wheat, nuts, and seeds. If your diet is low in whole grains, supplement with 100 to 400 IU of vitamin E per day.

Phytochemicals

Phytochemicals are substances found in fruits and vegetables that researchers believe may have cancer-fighting properties. Because they are natural antioxidants, phytochemicals have a detoxifying effect, helping the body eliminate harmful substances more efficiently. If you have a family history of cancer, or if you smoke, drink considerable amounts of alcohol or caffeine, or live in a polluted environment, it makes sense to up your intake of phytochemicals, either through eating more fruits and vegetables or by taking antioxidant vitamin supplements.

Calcium

The importance of calcium in preventing osteoporosis cannot be overstated. The recommended calcium intake for women over 35 is between 1,000 and 1,500 mg daily.

But calcium is tricky. It's not enough to simply get it into the body; there's also the problem of keeping it in. Certain drugs, such as tetracycline antibiotics, cholestryamine, and even Metamucil can interfere with calcium absorption. An excessive intake of caffeine, alcohol, or the phosphorus found in many processed foods and soft drinks can cause a woman to excrete calcium in her urine. Excessive protein—more than 40 grams a day (not an unusual amount in our society)—can also cause calcium deficiency and, ultimately, osteoporosis.

If you're concerned about maintaining calcium, limit your consumption of processed foods, protein, and caffeine. If you live in a cloudy climate with little natural exposure to sunshine, taking 400 IU of vitamin D daily will also aid in calcium absorption, as will taking a calcium supplement fortified with magnesium.

Note: You can probably meet your antioxidant requirements with a good multivitamin, but calcium is a bulky mineral and a daily dose just won't fit into a single pill. So prepare to supplement your multivitamin with three 500 mg calcium tablets a day, at least one of these being at bedtime.

Vitamin B_6

It has long been suspected that vitamin B_6 may function as a natural diuretic and, as a result, may help relieve PMS and perimenopausal symptoms, although this has not yet been proven. Taking it can't hurt, as long as you take care not to exceed 25 mg a day. Too much B_6 can cause tingling or burning sensations of the skin.

Iron

Nutritionists used to advise iron supplements for almost all women because it was believed that the very process of menstruation depleted iron. But ionized iron is now known to be an oxidant, one of the bad boys associated with increased cancer risk and heart disease. Unless you're anemic, back off from the iron supplements; you're probably getting all you need through your diet, and megadoses of this mineral are not recommended.

Step 2: Cut Fat

In the typical American diet, 37 percent of the calories come from fat. Ideally, less than 30 percent of your calories should come from fat. The following suggestions can help you reduce your fat intake.

1. Eat less visible fat. Either limit your use of all fat products, such as butter, oils, and salad dressings, or switch to the lowfat or nonfat varieties.

2. Eat your meat cooked as plainly as possible; broiling, steaming, poaching, grilling, or stir-frying are best. Trim visible fat, including poultry skins, before cooking; otherwise the fat is absorbed into the meat during the cooking process. Marinating in fat-free dressing or wine can add flavor without adding fat. Avoid deep-frying, casseroles, and heavy sauces —techniques capable of turning even innocent vegetables into caloric disasters.

3. Use lowfat or nonfat dairy products. The dairy industry has come a long way, offering a wider variety of lowfat cheeses, yogurts, sour creams, cottage cheeses, and imitation ice creams. Buy the new products in small amounts and taste test them; some will probably seem rubbery or bland, but others may strike you as being close in flavor to the original.

   Choose cheeses with fewer than 5 grams of fat per serving. If you're used to whole milk, gradually work your way down from 2 percent to 1 percent to 0.5 percent to nonfat. Let yourself adjust slowly to the other fat-free products as well, perhaps mixing fat-free sour cream with whole sour cream on your baked potato or combining reduced-fat and standard cheeses in your lasagna until you adjust to the differences in taste and texture.

4. Read labels. Thanks to the Nutritional Labeling and Education Act of 1990, nutritional information on labels is much more complete than it used to be.

   Nonetheless, manufacturers can still mislead you. "Cholesterol free" doesn't mean "fat free" and many products that proudly claim to have no cholesterol are loaded in fat. Another trick is basing calorie and fat estimates on a ridiculously small serving size. Does anyone really split a pint of frozen yogurt between six people? A good rule of thumb when looking at a label is to make sure there are no more than 2 to 3 grams of fat per 100 calories.

5. Educate yourself. Innumerable books on lowfat cooking are available, as are charts that allow you to calculate your fat intake down to the very last gram. Many hospitals and schools have affordable or free classes on lowfat cooking, how to shop for lowfat foods, and how to read labels.

6. Most fast food chains now have nutritional analysis available upon request, so if you eat fast food on a regular basis, ask to see the chart and study the fat content. There's usually one decent choice on the menu.

7. Snack on fruits, vegetables, plain popcorn, pretzels, rice cakes, and whole-grain crackers. Not only are high-fat foods so dense in calories that you can blow your whole food plan with one handful of peanuts, but there is increasing evidence that high-fat foods increase the levels of serotonin in the body. Serotonin works on the brain in a mood-altering way, often leading to a quick rush followed by depression and lethargy. Chocolate is the number one culprit.

Step 3: Eat More Fiber

Fiber aids elimination and cuts the risk of colon and rectal cancers. It's also important in weight control, because a high-fiber diet moves food more quickly through the digestive tract. Foods that are high in fiber tend to be nutritional bonanzas.

High-fiber foods include whole-grain breads and cereals, bran, fruits, vegetables, and beans, especially lima, navy, and kidney beans. But because these bottom-of-the-pyramid foods are so underrepresented in our diets, the average woman gets only 11 grams of fiber a day. She needs 20 to 30 grams for optimum health.

Begin with fruits and vegetables. Eat them raw, or steam or microwave them to maintain maximum fiber. After a couple of weeks, move on to high-fiber breads or cereals. Bread should have 2 to 3 grams of fiber per serving, and if you don't like the taste of whole grains, there are fiber-enriched white and rye breads on the market. Cereal manufacturers have jumped on the fiber bandwagon with both feet, so you'll have a huge selection there. Look for 5 grams per serving, but remember that the 1-ounce serving size listed on most cereal boxes is very small. If you're eating a whole bowl of cereal every morning, you're eating at least 2 servings and a fiber count of 3 grams per serving means you're actually eating closer to 6 grams of fiber.

Now for the beans. They're high in fiber, low in fat, and can form the base of many good soups, chilis, and Southwestern dishes.

Two words of warning: Don't introduce fiber all at once. If you go from 10 grams to 30 overnight, you may get sick. Start with the foods that are easier to digest, such as fruits and whole-grain breads, and add the beans last. Also, drink lots of water. Fiber creates bulk, and unless that bulk is kept softened by 8 to 10 cups of water daily, you'll become constipated.

Detoxifying the Body

For optimum health, it's not enough to get good things into your body—you'll also need to get the bad things out.

Eliminating Alcohol

There's no question that heavy drinking is bad for you, making you more vulnerable to cancer, heart disease, liver disease, diabetes, and, of course, alcoholism. For women, drinking also brings a less-publicized danger: Alcohol interferes with your body's ability to absorb calcium.

Because heavy alcohol use often causes premature menopause, stopping estrogen production an average of five years earlier than normal, there's a doubled risk for women who drink. The earlier you experience menopause, the more years your bones are weakened by estrogen depletion. If alcohol also compromises your body's ability to absorb calcium, you have twice the average risk for osteoporosis.

Moderate drinking brings more moderate risks, but as we saw in Chapter 6, regularly consuming more than one glass of wine can increase your chance of breast cancer. In addition, some women report that a couple of glasses of wine can trigger a hot flash. Two 3 ounce glasses of wine contain approximately 200 calories—not enough to blow your daily limit—but alcohol also releases inhibitions, resulting in the sort of what-the-hell attitude that can cause even the most fat-conscious woman to polish off a whole tray of nachos.

Drinking can also influence your sleep cycle. Some women report that a glass of wine helps them get to sleep, but they awaken five hours later. For women who suffer from insomnia or disrupted sleep, alcohol only makes the goal of a good night's rest more elusive.

Even taking all this into consideration, there is some evidence that one drink a day might be good for you. A well-publicized study released several years ago showed that, despite their high-fat diet, the French have a lower rate of heart disease than Americans. The theory is that red wine, which the French drink in abundance, increases the levels of good cholesterol (HDL) in the blood. In the final analysis, it seems that a drink on special occasions or when you're going out to dinner is a relatively harmless indulgence, and it's only when you're overimbibing on a regular basis that your health is compromised.

Eliminating Caffeine

In excessive amounts, caffeine can accentuate urinary stress incontinence, retard calcium absorption, and interfere with your ability to relax. If you're prone to insomnia or irritability, switch to decaffeinated coffee and soft drinks.

Coming off caffeine can leave you dragging, especially if you're hooked on your morning cup of java. Make the change slowly by having caffeinated coffee for your morning drink and decaf for the rest of the day or by mixing the two for a low-caffeine blend for the first few weeks. There are some low-caffeine coffees on the market that can also help you bridge the gap. Excedrin, which contains small amounts of caffeine, can both wean you off slowly and help you with your detox headache.

Eliminating Nicotine

No need to equivocate here: Every survey is in agreement that smoking is dangerous. Obviously, smoking brings a sharply heightened risk of lung cancer, and despite all the press about breast cancer, lung cancer remains the number one cancer killer of American women. In fact, smoking ultimately claims the life of 35 percent of the people who take up the habit, either through cancer or coronary disease. Would you fly an airline whose planes crashed one-third of the time? Considering how cautious we are in some areas of health care, our continuing tolerance of smoking is a case of a culture in collective denial.

Nicotine, much like alcohol, brings on an earlier menopause and limits calcium absorption. If a woman smokes and drinks, she'll likely be in estrogen depletion longer than normal, with fewer years to build up her bones and more years in which they'll be breaking down. Her heart will also be at risk years longer than normal—or necessary.

Most smokers are well aware of the facts and have tried to quit, but nicotine is highly addictive, more so than many of the so-called "hard" drugs we were warned about in college. Many women addicted to nicotine claim that it calms them, but as the effect of one cigarette wears off, they have to light another immediately or suffer the withdrawal jitters. Part of a smoking addiction is the ritual involved: When the phone rings or after the last bite of a meal, smokers have subconsciously programmed themselves to reach for the pack.

The subconscious, however, can always be reprogrammed, and many women find help in support groups or through hypnosis or biofeedback. Those who find the physical aspects of the addiction more overpowering than the psychological might try weaning themselves off nicotine with skin patches or gum.

Zyban (also sold as Wellbutrin, an antidepressant) is prescribed for some people who are having trouble kicking the habit. Patients begin the medication two weeks before they stop smoking and many people find it helps tame the cravings and agitation associated with nicotine withdrawal. Zyban doesn't substitute for nicotine, however, and adding patches or gum might make your efforts more effective.

Exercise is also an ally. Studies have shown that people who exercise are far less likely to resume smoking than sedentary former smokers. Exercise also helps counteract the weight gain that often accompanies giving up cigarettes. In her practice, Nancy has seen women who begin smoking again because they can't tolerate the weight gain. But remember: The 10 pounds you may gain by kicking a pack a day habit is much less than the 50 pounds' worth of extra work for your heart generated by smoking that pack of cigarettes. Smoking also ages the skin. Although some skin care treatments designed to offset the effects of time and sun damage actually seem to turn back the clock, the facial wrinkles caused by smoking are permanent.

For more information on giving up smoking, contact the American Cancer Society or the American Lung Association, listed in the Sources section in the back of this book

Stress Relief

The degree to which stress impacts our lives varies. We may all need the same amount of vitamins A and E, but how much R&R each woman needs depends on her lifestyle.

When you refer to the list of perimenopausal symptoms outlined in Chapter 3, you can't help but notice how many of them are worsened by stress. You may live the life of an Olympian, but if you continue to worry, you're putting yourself at risk for everything from colds to cancer. Even if you've never felt the need to learn stress-reduction techniques before, perimenopause is definitely the time to expand your horizons.

Several of the women we surveyed for this book mentioned that the effects of hormonal changes were intensified by life events. Change is inherently stressful, so even a happy event such as a marriage or a job promotion (or writing a book!) can take a toll on your nerves.

Just as many factors can cause stress, a variety of methods can alleviate it. Not everything on the list that follows will be your cup of tea, but keep an open mind. Eventually you'll find a stress-management technique that works for you.

Techniques for Managing Stress

Meditation   Classes in meditation and self-hypnosis will help you learn the basics, while various audiotapes can lead you through progressive relaxation exercises. If you're feeling unfocused, tense, or suffering from memory lapses, try one of the energizing routines. If insomnia is a problem, using a relaxation tape to help you get to sleep is far preferable to relying on pills or alcohol to make you drowsy.

Self-hypnosis not only helps people relax and control their anxiety but also counteracts some of the physical symptoms of perimenopause, including hot flashes. Because many of the symptoms of perimenopause are at least partially triggered by stress, self-hypnosis can intervene, breaking the maddening cycle of stress leading to a symptom that in turn leads to heightened stress and a heightened symptom.

Biofeedback If your stress level is so high that it is causing anxiety attacks or physical illnesses such as migraines or ulcers, you need more help than conventional meditation offers. Biofeedback teaches you how to use visualization and relaxation techniques to counteract physical problems and has proven exceedingly helpful in stress reduction. For more information on this technique, contact the Association of Applied Biofeedback, listed in the Sources section in the back of this book.

Aerobic Exercise It isn't necessary to exercise past the point of exhaustion or feel the celebrated "runner's high" to reap psychological benefits from exercise. Studies have shown that any regular aerobic activity releases endorphins, hormones that contribute to your overall sense of well-being. People who exercise are also more apt to describe themselves as being in control and to feel a greater sense of mastery in all areas of their lives.

Yoga and Tai Chi Chuan Yoga is a system of physical exercises and stretches combined with deep breathing and relaxation. Many women turn to yoga as they age for the flexibility benefits, but it's an undeniable stress-buster as well. After years of being eclipsed by aerobics, yoga is making its way back into the mainstream; your local exercise club or community college mostly likely has a course. *Yoga Journal* also has produced an excellent series of videotapes.

Tai chi chuan, an exercise discipline that originated in China, is also gaining popularity. Like yoga, there is an emphasis on breathing, body alignment, and flexibility, but tai chi is designed to stimulate as well as relax, and for that reason it is a good wake-up routine. The exercise of choice for the elderly in the Orient, many people claim that tai chi is one reason that the Chinese enjoy enviably good health as they age, with much lower rates of cancer and arthritis than Americans in the same age group.

Massage   Nothing is more pleasurable than a good massage, and women who schedule massages on a regular basis report that they rest better and that they feel their body release toxins more effectively. As with the other relaxation techniques mentioned in this chapter, it's worth going the professional route a few times to make sure you understand the basic techniques. Health spas and beauty salons often have a massage therapist on staff.

After you get a sense of what a good massage is all about—no jerking, pinching, or excessive pressure—you may want to buy one of the videotapes or books on massage and try it yourself. Aside from a relaxation technique, this can be an affectionate way to communicate with a friend or romantic partner.

Retreats and Spas   If you've ever thought about a spa vacation, perimenopause can be an excellent time to give it a try. The beauty of a spa or retreat is that you have the whole day simply to focus on yourself, exercising, reading, being pampered, or enjoying nature. Many spa guests are women traveling solo, making the experience almost like summer camp for adults. And because most spas focus on helping you instigate long-term changes in your health and teaching you relaxation techniques you can take with you, the benefits of a spa vacation can last far beyond your week in the sun.

Obviously, all this pampering doesn't come cheap, but many salons are beginning to offer "spa days," in which you can sample massages, facials, and other services for a more affordable price.

Saunas, Hot Tubs, and Whirlpool Baths   Relaxing after a workout is an important step in achieving the maximum benefits of exercise. Many health clubs offer saunas and hot tubs, while growing numbers of people are opting to install whirlpools or hot tubs in their homes. If you like the idea of massage, but can't see taking the time and money to regularly schedule appointments with a pro or you lack a suitable massage partner, 20 minutes in your whirlpool tub can be a quick and simple way to wind down before you go to bed.

Therapy and Support Groups   Menopause doesn't occur in a vacuum. It can hit in the midst of divorce, financial setbacks, retirement or work dislocation, children leaving home, parents growing more helpless, and all the other flotsam and jetsam of life.

Many women benefit from transition therapy during this hectic stage of their lives, and others find tremendous solace in joining a group of women who are going through similar disruptions. Carol, a young cancer patient thrown into early menopause, credits the women in her postcancer support group with "saving her emotional life" and helping her sort out which emotions were due to the illness, which to chemotherapy, which to her premature menopause, and which were just general life junk. "I had reached the point where I'd lost all perspective," she says, "and felt I was the only one who was going through this. My support group did more than any other single thing to bring my stress level down and teach me how to laugh again."

Speaking of laughter, you can employ a little self-therapy by taking in a funny movie, scheduling a weekend away, or just meeting a friend for lunch. Much of our tension is due to overwork, isolation from friends, and the frantic pace of our lives. Making a weekly date with yourself and using it specifically to hang out in a theater, museum, mall, or bookstore can go a long way toward reducing the treadmill feeling so familiar to women in midlife.

Menopause is the time of your life to take care of you. It's important to learn to say no to demands, and to set aside time for yourself. This may mean resetting your priorities and your standards about housekeeping, community service, and volunteering or how much time you spend doing social activities you really don't enjoy. Recognize that you can't do it all and expect to live to be 80. Even if you opt to handle your stress through the "head" method of group or individual therapy, don't forget that the mind-body connection is profound. You'll still benefit from exercise, relaxation tapes, massage, and the other methods mentioned here. The women who combat stress most effectively take a multilevel approach.

Attitude

The single key component in wellness is attitude. When you see that the changes you're making have an impact, the domino effect will begin to work for good instead of ill. In Chapter 3, we discussed how one problem can lead to another, but it's equally true that one positive change can lead to another. Exercise makes you less likely to smoke. Giving up smoking makes it easier to exercise. In making dietary changes you'll not only lose weight but your body will absorb more calcium and build bone and muscle mass, which in turn revs your metabolism and helps you keep the weight off. Utilizing relaxation techniques helps you get a good night's sleep so you don't need your morning shot of caffeine. Thanks to the positive domino effect, you'll find that once you make the first change all subsequent changes will be easier, resulting in a spiraling pattern of wellness.

9

Finding the Right Doctor

Nothing is easier than to accumulate facts, nothing is so hard as to use them.

—Oscar Wilde

Women are more likely to get their information on menopause from the news media or from friends than from a physician. We enter menopause much as we entered adolescence, with more "street knowledge" than hard facts.

Why don't women talk to their doctors? Sometimes it's just a lack of access. Many women entering perimenopause may not have seen their gynecologist or family doctor for several years, particularly if they have finished childbearing and have permanent contraception. Perimenopause sneaks up on them, and they valiantly try to ignore the symptoms. Even if they visit their doctor, the emphasis is on business as usual—Pap smears and breast checks—and they'll downplay any symptoms or menstrual irregularity.

Because we're trained to deny aging, and therefore menopause, for as long as we can, the symptoms are often pretty intrusive by the time a woman mentions them. That's part of the reason so many women are frustrated when they finally admit that "something's not right" and don't get much of a response from their doctor. Few gyne-cologists are menopause experts; many buy into the defi-nition of menopause as the cessation of menstruation and fail to connect the symptoms of a still-bleeding woman to hormone deprivation.

If you're one of the lucky few whose doctor recognizes the condition and uses the term *perimenopause,* your dis-cussions are still apt to focus on your short-term symp-toms. What you may get is a two-minute talk on hot flashes with little information on long-term health implications— and even less emphasis on midlife sexuality or the emo-tional side effects of entering menopause.

Since we wrote the first edition of this guide, more women have become members of HMOs and other man-aged care organizations, the structure of which tends to put pressure on physicians to see large numbers of pa-tients per day. Compounding the problem is the fact that many managed care health plans will not pay for specialty care without a referral from the patient's primary care physician, another speed bump in getting to the right doc-tor. In addition, insurance companies insist on discounted fees if specialists are to see their insured customers, a dis-incentive to the doctor to take on patients with complex medical conditions.

All these factors make it less likely that your doctor will want to take the time to talk with you about midlife changes. This makes it more vital than ever that you edu-cate yourself about your treatment options and be choosy about your doctor.

In the next chapter, we'll hear several women's indi-vidual stories about their passage into and through peri-menopause. Although their concerns and opinions vary widely, one striking commonality emerges from almost all of the stories: how awful their doctors were. The medical community's insensitivity toward menopausal women sur-faced again and again in the support groups we visited and among the women we interviewed. You can't assume that your longtime physician will be up on the latest meno-pause treatments or will even take your complaints seri-ously, but your chances of a successful dialogue improve if you approach the subject in the right way.

Schedule a Consultation

When you're climbing down from the stirrups after your annual Pap smear, it's hardly the best time to begin a dis-cussion on perimenopause. At best, your doctor has 20 minutes blocked out for your appointment, so he or she may behave as if there's no time for your questions, simply because there isn't. It's not fair to you or your doc-tor to try to sneak in a heavy discussion at the end of a rou-tine physical.

A far better strategy is to schedule an appointment for a consultation concerning your perimenopausal symp-toms. By asking the doctor to set aside time for a consul-tation, you allow him or her to focus on the problem and also signal that you really do consider this important. Don't expect your physician to take your complaints seri-ously if you treat them as peripheral.

A consultation also goes a long way toward reducing the inequity inherent in most doctor-patient discussions. It's hard to feel you're being treated as an equal when you're lying naked on a table, speaking up to someone who is fully dressed and clearly in a hurry. But if you meet over your doctor's desk, both sitting up, clothed, and with enough time to talk through the subject in detail, it's eas-ier to establish the feeling of a partnership.

Your doctor should be able to explain how HRT is dif-ferent for women in perimenopause than menopause; help you tally your individual risks for disease or side effects; and discuss the pluses and minuses of various treatments. He or she should not cheerlead for HRT or automatically reject it. During the consultation, you'll likely get a good idea of the depth of your doctor's interest in and knowledge about the field of perimenopause, HRT, and alternative treatments. Just as importantly, you'll discover how comfortable you feel discussing the issues with him or her.

In a busy menopause practice, registered nurses and nurse practitioners are often the ones who end up answering patient questions, giving out basic information, and in some cases handling follow-up visits for medication checks. So it's also important that you have a rapport with your physician's staff; hour for hour, you may be spending more time with them than you do with your doctor.

Prepare to pay as much or more for your initial consultation as you'd pay for an annual physical. It will take longer and represents a higher complexity of medical expertise and decision-making, both important factors in coding a visit for billing and insurance claims. This consultation may not be covered by your insurance, especially if you're going "out of the network" and not using a doctor included in your plan or if your primary care doctor won't give you a referral to a reproductive endocrinologist. But it is often still worth it to pay for a consultation out of your own pocket, even if you can afford only one visit with a specialist. The session will at least give you an outline of suggested care to take back to your regular doctor.

Is This the Right Doctor for You?

What's with all this "he or she" business? Does your doctor's gender matter? Many of the women we spoke with said they specifically looked for a female doctor because they found women physicians more empathetic. The more long term and complex the women's treatment—in other words, the more visits they had to schedule—the more apt they were to insist that a woman physician be their guide.

Amanda, who we'll meet in the final chapter, was an active professional when she entered perimenopause. She not only traveled widely in her job, but also held a rather high-profile position that required public speaking. She went to see her doctor (who happened to be male) when her periods had become so heavy that she was bleeding every day of the month. His response was a shrug and, "I realize this might be an inconvenience. . . ." Amanda snorts at the memory. "Inconvenience! No woman professional would have dismissed another's problems with a comment like that." Amanda ultimately found a female physician who appreciated the degree to which her symptoms were affecting her work and, although it took several changes of medication, her periods are now regular.

This to not to imply that all male physicians are clods and all female physicians saints; only that, everything else being equal, you might feel more comfortable with a woman. Nonetheless, from this point on we'll refer to the physician as "he," not because we're sexist, but to make it semantically easier to distinguish the doctor from the patient.

Issues of gender aside, how do you know if your doctor is the right person to take you through perimenopause and beyond? If he won't agree to a consultation or seems to find it a bizarre request, that's your first clue that something's wrong. Also, if his waiting room is full of pregnant women, that should tip you off that the obstetrical side of his practice is his emphasis and that nonsurgical gynecological patients might not get the same degree of attention.

Some physicians will make statements during the course of your evaluation and treatment that will send up red flags that they don't have the right degree of expertise or interest. The comments that follow were actually made to women we surveyed; if you hear remarks like these, climb down from that table and head for the nearest exit.

Top 10 List of Insensitive Physician Comments

10. "You're too young to be going through menopause."

9. "My wife takes these hormones and is doing just fine."

8. "Ask your friends what they use and let me know."

7. "Take this bag of hormone samples and see which one you like best."

6. "All women your age go through this—it's just something you have to put up with."

5. "Your only problem is that you're under too much stress."

4. "I don't start women on HRT until they haven't had a period for a year."

3. "I always . . ."

2. "I never . . ."

1. "I give up!"

What to Expect During an Office Visit

During your first visit, you can save your doctor a lot of time, and consequently save yourself a lot of money, if you bring a calendar or diary charting any menstrual irregularities you've experienced. Note such symptoms as hot flashes, sleep disturbances, mood swings, and headaches, and where they occur in your cycle. Are the symptoms more pronounced at some times of the month than others? On a separate sheet list other symptoms that may not be tied to hormonal fluctuations, such as joint aches, vaginal dryness, irritability, and memory lapses (see Figure 9.1).

Also be aware of your personal "misery index." How have these changes affected your quality of life? Do you miss days at work because of extremely heavy periods? Are

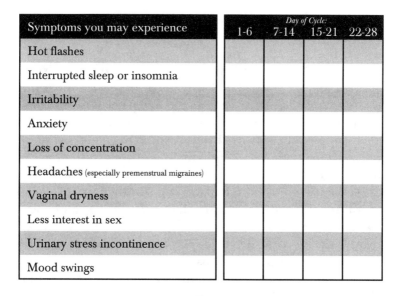

Symptoms you may experience	Day of Cycle:			
	1-6	7-14	15-21	22-28
Hot flashes				
Interrupted sleep or insomnia				
Irritability				
Anxiety				
Loss of concentration				
Headaches (especially premenstrual migraines)				
Vaginal dryness				
Less interest in sex				
Urinary stress incontinence				
Mood swings				

Figure 9.1 By keeping track of your symptoms and their timing during your menstrual cycle, you can help your doctor determine where you are in the menopausal process, as well as what therapies may be most helpful.

you less effective on the job because of mood swings or nervousness? Is your relationship with your family changing? Has your sex drive diminished? If your misery index is low, just talking with your doctor and realizing the stage of life you're entering may be adequate. However, if your work, relationships, or general self-esteem have begun to suffer, you need to discuss treatment alternatives.

The key word is *alternatives.* Be wary if your doctor claims he "always" treats his patients any one way and it's "always" effective. If your doctor either tries to ram HRT down your throat or, conversely, makes a blanket statement against it, recognize that he's more interested in selling a philosophy than in treating you as an individual.

Most doctors have a standard or pet regimen they try first, which is fine, but beyond that your physician should be flexible. The only thing worse than having a physician who pooh-poohs your symptoms is having a physician who uses a prefab treatment for every patient. A cartoon we saw showing a woman whose mouth has been taped shut with an Estraderm patch clearly illustrates that some doctors use HRT to silence a patient they perceive as a complainer. A physician truly committed to treating women at midlife won't simply throw HRT at his patients; he'll help you make the evaluation in light of your entire health history. He should also be well versed in combating symptoms via nutrition, exercise, and stress reduction. If a treatment doesn't work, the right doctor is willing to change the medication or the treatment, not argue that something's wrong with the patient.

A tuned-in doctor will use this time to begin screening a woman for cholesterol and breast cancer, if she isn't already having this done. Bone density tests should be considered for women at particular risk for osteoporosis. Contraceptive needs should be reevaluated. General health concerns regarding diet, nutrition, exercise, and smoking should be reassessed. Sometimes there are doubts about whether a woman is actually in menopause or not: FSH and estradiol tests may be helpful in making that determination.

If You Opt for HRT

Once a program of hormone replacement therapy is prescribed, you should receive instruction from the doctor or nurse in how and when to take the pills, apply the patch, and so on. Calendars on which to mark breakthrough bleeding and other symptoms are helpful. You definitely should not be handed a prescription and told, "Good luck. Come back in a year." A follow-up visit in two to four months is necessary to evaluate your initial response to therapy, check for side effects, and review your bleeding pattern.

The next visit should be anywhere from six to nine months after you begin HRT. Fine-tuning or even completely changing the medication is not uncommon in the first year of treatment and may be necessary again as you move through full-blown menopause.

Again, some practices have a nurse assigned to menopausal patients to answer their questions on the phone, deciding when they need to see the doctor versus making minor changes in their medication versus simple reassurance. So make an effort to meet all key members of the staff.

Try not to confuse a cautious response with a lack of concern. Sometimes it's appropriate for the doctor to hold off on HRT to see if the patient's misery index becomes intense enough to warrant therapy. The physician must also separate the patient who is clinically depressed from the patient with the mood swings of perimenopause. This is another good reason for an early follow-up visit; if the woman's hot flashes are gone but mood has not improved on HRT, she may need to be referred for treatment for depression. (See Chapter 10.)

At each follow-up visit, the patient and physician should review the reasons she is taking HRT and whether anything has happened in her health picture—an abnormal mammogram, a relative developing osteoporosis, and so on—that affects that decision or suggests a need for new testing.

When Is It Necessary to See a Specialist?

Ideally, if your gynecologist, internist, or family doctor is having difficulty managing your symptoms, he'll refer you to a specialist before you become so frustrated that you decide to take your business elsewhere. You'll probably need a menopause specialist or reproductive endocrinologist if:

- you're dissatisfied with the response you're getting from your doctor
- you're in perimenopause and trying to conceive
- your symptoms are unusually pronounced or aren't responding to conventional treatment
- you've had breast cancer or have a close family history of the disease and need someone versed in the latest on menopausal treatment

Many women find their specialist through word-of-mouth, and you're especially likely to be satisfied with your choice if you learn about a doctor from another woman. Sharing information about doctors is one of the key benefits of a menopause support group. For a list of reproductive endocrinologists or menopause specialists in your area, contact either the North American Menopause Society or the American Society for Reproductive Medicine, listed in the Sources section in the back of this book.

Seeing a specialist may require traveling to a medical center in another city, because women in suburban and rural areas don't always have easy access to specialized care. The cost can also be prohibitive. But if you have a good relationship with your gynecologist or family physician, there is no reason to completely transfer your medical care to the specialist; many are available for diagnostic and planning consultations only. Most reproductive endocrinologists don't aim to provide ongoing gynecologic care, but rather, they aim to get you settled on the proper regimen and then refer you back to your regular physician.

Finally, the term *specialist in menopause* is not a synonym for *specialist in hormone replacement therapy.* A specialist should be equally able to tailor a plan of management for the woman who doesn't want to take hormones, focusing on increased calcium, vitamin and herbal therapy, a lowfat diet, exercise, and monitoring for heart disease, osteoporosis, and breast cancer.

10

Psychology, Sexuality, and Perimenopause

The empty nest may actually be a love nest.

—Andrew Greeley

Let's forget for a moment about how perimenopause affects your body and focus on how it affects your mind. Even the women we surveyed who claimed to know nothing about menopause didn't hesitate to venture theories in this area—that menopause is a factor in mental illness, that it instantly makes a woman less sexual, that it is the first step in the descent into old age.

It's undeniable that hormones have an impact on both mood and sexuality, as any woman who has gone into sudden estrogen withdrawal can attest. But we are more than our hormones, and it is equally undeniable that our moods are influenced by many factors, not the least of which are our expectations. Menopause is often a self-fulfilling prophecy: A woman who believes it marks the end of youth will be more apt to blame every sexual slow-down and memory lapse on menopause than a woman who has a more positive mindset. In this chapter, we'll try to separate the problems that can accurately be attributed to menopause from those that cannot, and offer suggestions on how to deal with both.

Several of the women with whom we spoke mentioned that they weren't aware of how much their personalities had changed during perimenopause until someone else pointed it out or they looked at themselves in retrospect. "My kids kept telling me that I was edgy," they said, or "I see now that I was becoming antisocial." During the time in which the changes are happening, it can be tough to be objective about your own condition.

Does Perimenopause Cause Depression?

Contrary to myth, menopause doesn't cause depression.

We muddy the water in these discussions with our tendency to use the term *depression,* which is a specific and serious illness, as if it meant "in a bad mood" or "a little down." Estrogen deprivation can trigger a bad mood or sap your energy, but it does not bring on full-scale clinical depression (see Figure 10.1).

Depression is twice as common in women as in men, which is possibly the root of the misconception that menopause and mental illness are synonymous terms. But separate studies in the United States, England, and Sweden have all shown that women are no more prone to have their first bout of depression during menopause than at any other time.

This is not to say that estrogen, or a lack of it, doesn't affect your mood. When estrogen levels fall from their high during pregnancy, for example, 50 to 70 percent of women experience a mild, transient depression over the first 10 days after delivery. Ten to 20 percent develop a significant depression, and a tiny number—less than one-tenth of 1 percent—develop major psychosis.

Likewise, when estrogen levels drop during perimenopause, many women experience mood swings, and 65 percent of the women attending menopause clinics report feeling mildly depressed. Often these moods are linked

Perimenopause	Depression
Irregular periods	Feelings of worthlessness
Hot flashes, night sweats	Hopelessness, thoughts of suicide
Loss of concentration, memory loss	Difficult concentrating or making decisions
Weight gain	Unintentional weight gain or loss (≥5%), increase or decrease in appetite
Insomnia, poor sleep quality	Insomnia, with early A.M. wakening, inability to fall back to sleep
Fatigue	Fatigued, no energy
Irratibility, mood swings	Irritability, anger
Vaginal Dryness	

Figure 10.1 Perimenopause vs. Depression.

to another symptom, as in a case where hot flashes are keeping a woman from getting restful sleep.

Hormonal moodiness often involves feelings of lethargy, a lack of concentration, less interest in sex, and perhaps a decreased desire to socialize. HRT helps most women troubled with hormonal mood swings, because it relieves the underlying symptoms and because estrogen has a mood-altering effect on the brain. Specific receptors for estrogen are located in the limbic forebrain, the area that is responsible for our emotions. By stimulating serotonin production and yielding higher levels, estrogen acts similarly to the antidepressant Prozac.

It's important to remember that we're talking about using HRT to treat relatively minor depression and mood swings, not true despair. A woman who enters her doctor's office with thoughts of suicide or a complete inability to function is not suffering from hormonal depression and should not be immediately started on HRT in lieu of anti-depressants. Clinical depression is a life-threatening condition that requires psychiatric evaluation and therapy. HRT may help the woman feel better physically and in turn respond better to the antidepressant therapy.

Are Mood Swings Worse When Menopause Is Abrupt?

Usually the answer is yes. Women who undergo a rapid menopause, whether natural or medically induced, are at higher risk for depression than women who undergo menopause gradually. Their estrogen withdrawal is sudden, similar to what women experience after childbirth, leading to a hormonal crash. Some women who have gone through an abrupt menopause also report that their sex drive decreases dramatically; they may benefit from the addition of testosterone to their HRT regimen.

Is It All Hormonal?

As we've seen, many of life's stresses hit during perimenopause. A woman in her 40s may be experiencing kids moving out, kids moving back in, the responsibility of caring for aging parents, divorce, job loss or relocation, loss of friends, mixed feelings about growing older, and, as one woman put it, "a real resentment that my body suddenly seems to be turning on me." (See Figures 10.2a and 10.2b.)

Several of the women we interviewed specifically mentioned feeling out of control, as if their bodies had an agenda of their own. A 40-year-old woman who is in perimenopause may have a harder time with this control issue than a woman in her 50s, because the younger woman is dealing with an array of symptoms she didn't expect for another 10 years. No one wants a hot flash in the middle of a sales presentation, irregular periods while on a business trip, or to be facing divorce as the biological clock is ticking audibly.

An interesting statistic to ponder: Wealthier women report more menopausal symptoms than poorer women, no matter what country they live in. It seems paradoxical. Why would women with good nutrition, more education, and better access to health care have the most problems?

At first glance, this fact would seem to lend credence to the theory that women are just bitching, that the more money a woman has, the more leisure time she has to obsess about her symptoms. But this statistic more likely means that feeling good is a lower priority for people with low incomes. Poor women will typically suffer much longer than middle-class women before they seek medical help, and, in the presence of a doctor, often downplay the intensity of their symptoms. A hot flash may seem like a minor complaint compared to living in a dangerous neighborhood with the sound of gunfire outside the apartment window or making sure your family has enough to eat.

Perimenopausal depression may also be tied to a woman's expectations about aging. In cultures such as China, where the elderly are honored, few menopausal symptoms are reported. This could be because of differences in the Chinese diet and lifestyle—or it could be because Chinese women are proud to grow older. In the United States, lesbians are less troubled by menopausal symptoms than heterosexual women, and lesbian couples report no decline in libido or frequency of sexual activity.

We could speculate for days on why these differences exist, but in the meantime it's beyond question that menopause is doubly rough on women who live in a culture that is both male-dominated and youth-oriented. From the anxious articles on how to understand our husbands that

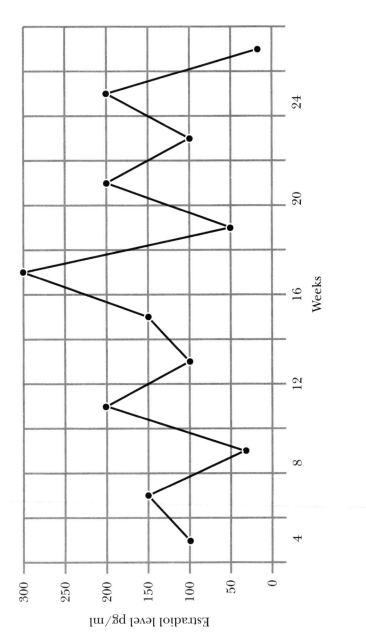

Figure 10.2a Variation in estradiol levels in perimenopause.

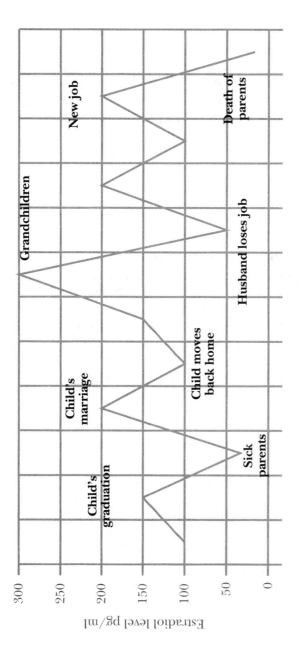

Estradiol level pg/ml

fill women's magazines to the sensationalized media reports on how few suitable men there are out there, it's obvious that our society equates a woman's self-worth with her ability to attract and hold a man. If a woman is indifferent to male perceptions of her, menopause may be inconvenient, but it probably isn't scary. On the other hand, if a woman feels she is competing for male attention with younger, more "hormonally advantaged" women, her fears about aging may become strong enough to literally make her sick.

Plastic Surgery

Now you may be asking, "So, assuming I'm not a lesbian in Beijing, should I visit a plastic surgeon? Is that your point?"

We're describing, not prescribing. Assuming that they can afford it, perimenopause is indeed a time when many women resort to plastic surgery. Common procedures include an abdominoplasty, or tummy tuck, which removes the loose skin from previous pregnancies or weight loss, and breast reconstruction. Women may also opt to have a face-lift, skin peels, or collagen injections to plump out facial wrinkles.

Liposuction has become the most common plastic surgery procedure in the United States among both women and men. Liposuction is not a cure for general obesity—an average of eight pounds is sucked out in a standard procedure—nor is it a substitute for diet and exercise. But because body fat distribution is largely hereditary, some otherwise fit women have pads of fat on their hips, thighs, or abdomens. Liposuction is used to remove the fat cells from these isolated places and improve the body's contours.

Many women find the idea of plastic surgery offensive, the result of unrealistic and sexist cultural demands that 50-year-olds look like 30-year-olds. They matter-of-factly point out that most men do not feel a corresponding pressure to hide their sags and bags, and assert that America has gone overboard in its worship of youth. Other women just as matter-of-factly point out that when they look better they feel better—so why not? One woman we interviewed, who has had four separate reconstructive procedures and is not yet 50, argued that the emphasis on the mind-body connection is usually given to how we can use our minds to improve our bodies. "But it works both ways," she says. "If you improve your body, it helps your mental attitude."

Because you'll bring your own value judgments to the issue, like so many of the topics we've discussed, cosmetic surgery remains a deeply private choice. Two things are certain: As we baby boomers move through middle age, plastic surgery is going to continue to be big business, and our society's attitude toward aging women is going to remain a hot topic.

Talking to Your Partner

Without getting into the issue of the male midlife crisis, it's worth mentioning that if your partner is having his own troubles adjusting to aging, this will influence how well you cope. If your husband dreads the thought of getting older, you may even wonder whether you should try to hide your complaints from him.

Yet a woman in menopausal transition needs to be open with her partner about her symptoms and how they're affecting her emotions, energy level, and sexual interest. Just as many women wait to see their doctors until the symptoms have become unbearable, they often wait to broach the subject with their partners until they're at the emotional breaking point.

Men certainly have no intrinsic understanding of menopause, so an explanation of just what a hot flash is may be called for, along with telling him what you're doing to address the problem. We've already discussed that women don't like feeling out of control. Well, no big surprise, but men hate it, too. If your husband seems indifferent to your symptoms, it may be because he feels helpless and is wondering, "Why are you telling me this if I can't do anything about it?"

As described in books like *Men Are from Mars, Women Are from Venus* by John Gray, women tend to make decisions while talking, using their friends or spouse as sounding boards while mentally running through the alternatives or simply venting. Men, in contrast, tend to speak only after the decision is made, take conversations more literally, and if you say, "I'm going crazy," may actually think, "My god, she's going crazy." An unemotional, results-oriented man will respond better to a conversation that basically says, "Here's what's going on with me, here's what I'm doing to combat it, and here's how you can help."

Also express what's positive about this time of life— no more need for birth control, no more periods or PMS. If you're instituting changes in your diet, starting to exercise, or learning stress-management techniques, invite him to participate. Then the focus moves from your menopause (that is, your "problem") into the broader sphere of what you both can do to make the coming years as terrific as possible. Aging isn't just about the negatives; it's also about travel, leisure, new hobbies, and more time to enjoy each other.

Frequency of Sexual Activity

And now you may be muttering, "Okay, okay. We'll take up golf, but our sex life is over, right?"

Different, maybe. But not over.

There is an age-related decline in the frequency of intercourse for both men and women, but menopausal women decrease their sexual activity more than men of the same age. In one study, 7 percent of women between the ages of 45 and 50 stated that they had "no interest in sex." This increased to 20 percent for 51- to 55-year-olds and to 31 percent by ages 56 to 60. Although many authors (and many husbands) attribute this decline in interest to changes in male function and behavior, studies haven't borne this out. Sexual frequency is tied more to the woman's interest level than to the man's, with little connection to either the male's age or level of interest or ability.

Just as most heart disease studies have focused on male subjects, so have most studies on mature sexuality, so the question of why older women lose interest in sex has never been fully addressed. Much has been made of the differences in male arousal time that come with age; it takes a man 3 seconds to get an erection at age 18, 20 seconds at age 45, and 5 minutes or more at age 75. But, let's face it, among all the complaints women have about men, "They're too slow sexually," doesn't usually make the top 10 list. How many women really care about this slowdown, unless they have a train to catch?

Men earnestly believe that women change in response to their changes—after all, our whole sexuality exists in response to theirs, right? But most women say that their lack of interest has more to do with what's going on inside them than what their partners are doing. Some women report that menopause doesn't bring on any decline in desire, while others confess that they're playing the myths about menopause to their own benefit, using them as an excuse to forgo sexual activity after what may have been years of indifference.

Studies show that rates of sexual activity fall steadily for both men and women from the ages of 20 to 40, but after 40, the decline becomes more dramatic. One study reported a decrease from 59 "episodes" per year at age 38 to 26 a year by age 50. In other words, by her late 40s a woman may be having sex less than half as often as she was at the beginning of her 40s. (It's important to remember that these statistics are based on some nonexistent "average" man and woman; some couples have sex rarely or never, while others, especially if their level of general marital satisfaction is high, have sex as often as they ever did.)

In this chapter, much as in the chapter on fertility, we may seem to be making the false assumption that every perimenopausal woman is in a relationship. We realize that women may go through years without a suitable partner, or even an unsuitable one, and sometimes the frequency of sex declines through lack of opportunity. If you aren't currently in a sexual relationship, and even if you have no plans to have one in the future, read on. Your vaginal health is still important, and most of the benefits of sexual stimulation, such as increased glandular and blood activity in the pelvic region, can be just as easily achieved through masturbation as they can through intercourse. Stimulation and orgasm, not the mere presence of a partner, are what keep your vagina healthy.

Physical Changes in the Genitals

When ovarian function ceases, you lose both estrogen and testosterone. As we've discussed, the loss of testosterone can dampen your desire for sex, but the loss of estrogen can actually affect your physiology. The following descriptions are not designed to terrify you. Just as with any other symptom, some women report the condition to a much greater degree than others and some women are completely unaffected.

The first changes you're apt to notice are in the outer genitals. Pubic hair thins and the labia loses fat tissue, meaning your vaginal lips become less full and less responsive to touch. Inside, the walls of the vagina thin and become more fragile as a result of the decreased blood supply. If the vagina is not stimulated through sexual play or masturbation, the diminished circulation will eventually affect the nerves and glands.

As the nerves lose function, there is less sensation during sex, and as the glands lose function, there's less lubrication. Needless to say, many women at this point are avoiding intercourse, thinking, "Why bother?" But abstinence accelerates the cycle of deterioration. The phrase "use it or lose it" may sound crass, but it's true.

If the early warning signs go untreated, the vagina will become smaller and less elastic, a condition known as vaginal atrophy. If a woman with vaginal atrophy attempts to have intercourse, she will find that, between the decreased lubrication and decreased elasticity, her vagina doesn't stretch to accommodate the man's penis as it used to do. At best, she feels nothing. At worst, she feels pain. In the very worst-case scenario, the walls of the vagina can tear during intercourse.

As if all this weren't enough, the acid base–balance of the vagina also changes, and the higher pH level makes it more susceptible to infections. An atrophied vagina is much more likely to become inflamed and to develop itching, discharge, and seemingly endless minor infections. Having vaginitis 40 weeks of the year can profoundly depress what's left of your sex drive.

Even if the vagina doesn't deteriorate completely, once estrogen depletion has begun to alter a woman's physiology, her response to sexual stimulation becomes muted. Besides the loss of skin receptivity, there's also less preorgasmic muscle tension and a delay in the reaction time of the clitoris, making a woman only half as likely to have an orgasm as she used to be.

Twenty-one percent of premenopausal women report that they have an orgasm every time they have sex, but only 10 percent of perimenopausal women climax every time. Menopause is only part of the reason. As a woman ages, her general health may decline (as may her partner's) and she is more likely to be taking medications, such as antihypertensives or even antidepressants like

Prozac, that inhibit sexual response.

After reading this laundry list of miseries, you may feel like popping a Prozac yourself, but take heart. Even if things are changing down below, the brain remains the chief sexual organ. Happily married and newly married women report that they enjoy sex as much at midlife as they ever did, and the previously cited reports about lesbians and women who live in cultures that celebrate aging only serve to emphasize that attitude is everything. If physiology were the sole component of sexuality we would all crave exactly the same amount of sex, and lose interest at the same time and at the same rate. Obviously, we don't.

Attitude also influences how women react to the physical changes; women who are essentially uninterested in sex will welcome an excuse to terminate their sex lives, and women who want to have sex will find a way to overcome the physical barriers.

How to Combat These Changes

HRT increases vaginal lubrication and reverses the thinning of the vaginal walls, relieving painful intercourse. If lack of lubrication and/or decreased vaginal sensation are your only symptoms, you may just require an estrogen cream to make sex fun again.

If you're trying to avoid HRT, start with an over-the-counter lubricant, such as Replens or Astroglide. Although it will not reverse thinning of or damage to the vaginal walls, a lubricant will make sex more comfortable, and because sex increases the blood supply to the area, you'll get the cycle turning once more in a more positive direction.

The key is not to wait too long before seeking intervention. Your doctor can test for vaginal dryness and atrophy, but by the time problems show up in a routine exam, they're pronounced. Only you know how much you naturally lubricate, how much you think or fantasize about sex, and how sex usually feels to you, so you will obviously be the first one to notice any changes. Don't convince yourself that it's all in your head and that desire will return on its own in a few months. If you avoid sex or masturbation altogether, you'll lose whatever elasticity and response you have left.

Even if you still feel as mentally interested in sex as ever and have noticed no pain or physical changes in your vagina, it may be taking you longer to become aroused or reach orgasm. Estradiol levels affect your whole central nervous system and influence nerve transmission, including the responses that contribute to sexual arousal. Estrogen replacement increases the blood flow to the pelvic area, awakens the receptor zones in the pudendal nerve, and can restore what the scientists refer to as "clitoral and vaginal vibration." In other words, estrogen can not only keep sex from being uncomfortable but can also restore a woman's ability to feel desire and pleasure.

Will Your Sex Life Be the Same?

Here's a variation on an old joke: A woman tells her doctor that she hasn't had an orgasm since menopause. Her doctor changes her medication, adds testosterone, and advises the use of lubricants. After months without improvement, she happens to mention that she never had an orgasm before menopause either.

HRT can't correct a problem that existed before menopause and this may be a good time to rethink your entire approach to sex. Only 20 percent of premenopausal women always experience orgasm, with about 60 percent sometimes coming to climax, and the remaining 20 percent having never had an orgasm. Obviously there are a lot of women out there who aren't reaching their full pleasure potential even before hormone withdrawal becomes an issue.

There are innumerable books on the market dealing

with the subject of midlife sexuality. *Sex Over 40* by Saul Rosenthal, M.D., provides information on the effects of menopause and male hormonal changes, common drugs that may affect sexuality, as well as intercourse positions for people who suffer from osteoporosis and joint problems. Although it doesn't focus specifically on any age group, *For Each Other: Sharing Sexual Intimacy* by Lonnie Barbach, Ph.D., does an excellent job of addressing the issues of diminished desire and the powerful effect the mind has on sexuality.

We spoke to women who changed partners, changed attitudes, and even changed their sexual orientation during this time of their lives. Although your transition might be less dramatic, it's important to keep an open mind. Many women we talked to pointed out that if you're looking for a new partner in this stage of life, the old rules no longer apply. You're less likely to be looking for a man to father your children or to give you social acceptability or financial security. Your primary requirement in a midlife relationship may just be "the pleasure of his company"—a factor frequently mentioned by women who ended up with a younger man, a man of a different race or religion, another woman, an unemployed artist, or someone they would never have considered a likely partner in their youth.

Because the focus is on how the other person makes them feel, women in midlife may make more adventurous choices than they made 25 years earlier. If you do seek a new sexual partner, remember to be vigilant about birth control and to use a condom if there is the slightest chance of exposure to a sexually transmitted disease.

Even if you're in a long-term relationship or marriage, medical conditions may force you to look for new ways to express your sexuality. The standard missionary position is a literal pain for women suffering from osteoporosis or vaginal atrophy; if the woman is on top she can control the depth of penetration and won't have to support her partner's weight. If the man has back or joint problems of his own, rear entry or side-by-side positions can keep you from hurting him. If you've noticed a slowdown in sexual response time, try oral sex, mutual masturbation, or a vibrator: During menopause you may require a more direct stimulation of the clitoris in order to reach orgasm.

And, of course, the statistics don't reveal it all. Frequency is not the only component of sexual satisfaction, and some women report that they're doing it less but enjoying it more. Sexuality flourishes for many women in their 50s and 60s, especially when they're willing to be creative. Menopause marks the end of your reproductive life, but the best years of your sexual life may still be ahead.

11

Talking with
Other Women

Too much agreement kills a chat.

—Eldridge Cleaver

Do you need a support group to help you through peri-menopause? At first the question may seem ridiculous. You're busy. You have friends. Do you really want to drive across town to hang out with a group of strangers when all you have in common is menstrual irregularity?

A support group doesn't have to be a formal organization associated with a hospital or clinic; we spoke with one group that evolved out of a bunch of high school friends that had promised to stay in touch after their twenty-fifth reunion. If you would describe your peri-menopausal experience as "typical," a network of friends may be all you need. Women with more specialized problems, however, such as those experiencing premature menopause or severe symptoms, will probably benefit from joining a focused group. If you're having a difficult time in menopause, you need to be around other women whose experiences mirror yours, not well-meaning but clueless friends assuring you that you're overreacting.

Benefits of a Support Group

Whether you opt to join an organized group or just be more open with friends, don't underestimate the importance of female bonding. Women who talk to other women do much better than those who go through this passage silently and alone. One of the key benefits of a group is shared information—the name of a sympathetic doctor, a debate on patches versus pills, or techniques on fighting sleeplessness. Women can also lobby collectively for changes in the health-care system with more authority than we can muster as individuals.

Many hospitals and women's clinics offer support groups, which are often made up of women who share a specific medical condition such as premature menopause, cancer, or infertility. If your needs are more general, you might check the Internet. Some sites are listed in the Sources section in the back of this book. Or look for a group whose roots are in a local women's organization, church, synagogue, or community center. A large city will likely have more than one group, with origins as diverse as the Junior League, a Catholic parish, or the local chapter of the National Organization of Women, making it easy to find one that fits your personal style.

Once you get through the door, you'll probably find you have more in common with these women than hot flashes. Women who tackle menopause head-on tend to be dynamic, proactive, interesting people who don't take aging lying down. "So many of the questions that come up in group," explains one woman, "revolve around a single concern: 'Is this normal?' We have a speaker every month, but often we answer that question before the expert even shows up. The answer is usually 'Yes, it's normal. I'm going through it too.'"

If you would like to start your own perimenopause support group, it can be as simple as finding a group of friends, taking turns meeting in each other's homes, and picking a discussion topic each month. For information on how to start a group or find an existing one, contact a women's clinic or hospital in your area or write to the North American Menopause Society, listed in the Sources section in the back of this book.

The Women's Stories

Every woman's transition into menopause is different, and nothing illustrates this more powerfully than the stories of the individual women we interviewed. We selected several women who went through the change, some smoothly, some not, and asked them what they would like to say to other women about their experiences.

Claudia

"Who was this person who was always crying, tired all the time? I was willing to do anything it took to get my old self back."

Claudia, an attractive, confident woman who used to be a fashion model, is the antithesis of the menopausal granny. She and her husband travel extensively for their import-export business and have two college-age sons. Claudia has lived on four continents.

"We'd moved with the kids nine times in our marriage and I thought I could handle change," she says wryly. But she was unprepared when, at 50, her periods suddenly stopped. "Within four months I went from being completely regular to having no bleeding at all. I felt like I had PMS all the time. I was tired, bloated, crying over anything, and anxious about ridiculous things." Although Claudia's everyday life was stressful enough to stop most women in their tracks, she never once felt that her changes in attitude were connected to anything but her hormones.

"I enjoy a fast pace," she says, "assuming I can get a good night's rest. But once I went into menopause, I had night sweats so bad that I was waking up dripping wet and unable to go back to sleep. It went on night after night, and I haven't felt anything like that level of exhaustion since my boys were babies. Within six weeks, my nerves were so ragged I was unable to work. I've always been appearance-conscious, but suddenly I was fighting a losing battle. I was too bloated to wear half my clothes, my skin and hair were dry, and I had bags under my eyes."

Claudia's longtime doctor described her complaints as "typical" and advised her to "tough it out." A second doctor put her on an estrogen skin patch, which she has used for five years with great success. "Within six weeks on estrogen, the hot flashes stopped, I was resting better and had my energy back," she says. "I resent even those few months I felt so bad, because it wasn't necessary.

"The thing is, my mother's life was predictable. She died in the same town she was born in. She expected to age at a certain rate, expected to die at a certain age, and, frankly, nothing much was required of her after menopause. She ended up living with two of her sisters. After lunch, they would all go lie down and pull the shades.

"But my life is unpredictable. I work. I travel. My siblings and I all live in different countries. The society I'm in happens to be preoccupied with youth, which is regrettable in many ways, but in another way it is good for me. I couldn't go into a bedroom at noon and pull the shades even if I wanted to. There's too much I'm expected to do."

Annie

"As long as I can avoid doctors and drugs, I will. My past experiences have all been bad."

Annie, a 46-year-old teacher with a teenage daughter, has been in perimenopause for at least eight years. "My body's always been off the normal pace," she shrugs. "I started having my periods at the age of nine and was skipping periods and having hot flashes by my late 30s. I still have periods sometimes, but they're irregular and very heavy and sometimes go on for a month at a time."

Although this menstrual roller coaster has drained her energy, Annie is reluctant to consider HRT. "I'm extremely phobic about drugs. I have a history of reactions, bad side effects. I won't even take an aspirin unless I'm absolutely desperate."

She has even more reservations about doctors. "No one has ever talked to me," she says flatly. "It's just 'Do you want this pill or not?' No explanations, no options, just a prescription. My doctor will not acknowledge my fears or even answer my questions." Twice worn down by periods that lasted for weeks, Annie got a prescription for HRT, but never had it filled. "I kept thinking I'd give it another day or two, and both times I stopped bleeding on my own.

"I can handle short-term symptoms like hot flashes, even the marathon periods if I have to. But there's a lot of heart disease in my family and I do wonder sometimes about the long-term effects. I'll be living a very long time without estrogen . . . and it's not like I enjoy wearing a pad every day of my life. I know it must seem like stubbornness, but it's really more a lack of information. I won't take anything until I have to, and I'll never take anything I don't understand. And so far I can't find anyone who can explain estrogen to me."

Amanda

"I'm using a combination of traditional medical solutions, like estrogen, along with alternative remedies like acupuncture and stress reduction. I pick and choose among everything that's available."

"When I went to my gynecologist, I was 44, about to be married, and pretty sure I was going into menopause," says Amanda. "It was not exactly the greatest time to be losing interest in sex and having vaginal dryness. He looked at my chart, not at me, and totally laughed off the idea of menopause. I asked him about estrogen, and he said 'You're too young.' He seemed insulted by my questions, like the very fact I was interested in my health care meant I was doubting his expertise or judgment.

"I told him about the vaginal dryness and he said, 'You're depressed.' I said I was a therapist and I'd know if I was depressed, thank you very much." She bristles at the memory. "When I told him about my menstrual problems, all he could say was that he'd do a D and C. Evidently that's his standard cure."

Wary of surgery and furious that her doctor didn't seem to trust her opinions about what was happening in her body, Amanda searched out a new gynecologist, a younger woman. "My new doctor is the first person I ever heard use the term *perimenopause*," she says. "We had a long interview in which she asked a lot of questions about my medical history and laid out all the options. Finding the right physician is so important because, believe me, this is a long-term relationship. It took me four changes of medication before I found the combination that worked. If you don't have faith in your doctor, you'll never get through the process."

Although HRT relieved many of her symptoms, her experience with her first doctor demonstrated to Amanda the need to take full responsibility for her own medical care. As a therapist, she was well aware of the effect stress can have on physical problems, and she began seeking alternative remedies as well as conventional treatment. Acupuncture has helped with her menstrual cramps, and she uses a variety of self-relaxation techniques to cope with the demands of everyday life. "I don't have an agenda when it comes to health care," she says. "I tell my M.D. about the acupuncturist and my friends at the health food store about the estrogen. I'll use whatever works."

Lynn

"Menopause was a breeze."

"I'm not really sure when menopause happened," says Lynn, a 49-year-old writer with children ages 11 and 9. "I was on birth control pills, and at some point my hormones must have just gradually tapered off." Now off the Pill, Lynn remembers "a couple of hot flashes and some vaginal dryness, which I handled with a drugstore lubricant." She is not eager to take HRT. "I enjoy not having periods."

Although she feels great and is able to reconcile the demands of job and family with enviable ease, Lynn occasionally worries about aging. "There's lots of osteoporosis in my family," she says. "My mother had the hump. My sister lifts weights and is absolutely religious about taking calcium. I keep meaning to buy a bottle.

"Some things about aging have been tough for me. Both my parents are dead, which has brought me face-to-face with my own mortality. But menopause was easy. I don't mourn the loss of my ability to bear children and my sex life is better than ever. I think that if you don't have many physical symptoms, it's easy not to think about the emotional issues, and since I never had this big bang, this moment of 'Oh, I'm in menopause,' I don't really feel all that changed. It's okay to say that, isn't it? That for me menopause was no big deal?"

Debbie

"Over the past year I've been diagnosed with cancer, had chemotherapy, and gone into menopause. I had to let go of the control issue. Things I never would have predicted were happening to my body, and all I could do was respond to them. Feeling powerless was the worst part."

Debbie was 33 when chemotherapy following lymphatic cancer destroyed her ovaries and threw her into an immediate menopause. "My ovaries were dead by the second chemo treatment," she says. "I had the whole package within two weeks—hot flashes, vaginal dryness, insomnia, depression."

Debbie's doctor nagged her until she overcame her lethargy and joined a hospital support group designed for women in chemically induced menopause. "After the meeting," she remembers, "for the first time in a long time I considered myself lucky. I have a son, but two of the women in the group had gotten cancer while they were in their 20s and single. On top of everything else, they were dealing with this tremendous anger that they'd never have children."

Debbie's new friends helped her wade through the arduous process of sorting out the cancer-related symptoms from those related to stress and menopause. "I was tired, weepy, and had horrible memory loss, the kind where you would start writing a check and literally forget your own name. At first I blamed it all on the chemo. But after the chemo was wrapped up and I was still having symptoms, I had to say 'Wait a minute. . . .'"

The fact that so many of her symptoms seemed interconnected made it hard for Debbie to pinpoint what was causing what, much less how to tackle the problem. "Having cancer is so overwhelming that you focus completely on it," she says. "I'm not sure I would have connected any of the symptoms to a loss of estrogen if it hadn't been for the other women. Collectively we were having so many of the same things happen to us that as time passed we kept sharing information and finding answers as a group."

Working closely with her team of doctors and bouncing ideas off her support group, Debbie has begun a combination of HRT and natural remedies. "If you're in a premature menopause," she concludes, "you have to work to get over the control issue. If I hadn't been able to come to terms with the fact that things were happening to me beyond my control, I never would have been able to move on. My sense of isolation was heavy—not too many women in their 30s have to deal with what I'm dealing with—but my support group made all the difference."

Peggy

"I found women reluctant to band together and accept the label 'menopausal.'"

"I disappointed myself in how I reacted to aging," admits Peggy, an energetic 51-year-old executive. "I thought I was above being bothered by it, but I discovered in my forty-ninth year that I was bothered big-time about it."

Peggy's epiphany came on a vacation with her daughter, when a man approached their table in a restaurant and asked if he could join them. "He was maybe 10 years younger than me, easily 20 years older than my daughter," Peggy recalls, "and it took me half the meal to realize it was her he was interested in, not me. I thought, 'This is it. The torch has passed on to the next generation. I'm invisible.'"

When Peggy first began experiencing menopausal symptoms at age 45, she attributed them to stress. "I called it a malaise," she says. "My job is so intense that I connected the insomnia and exhaustion to work. All of a sudden I didn't want to go out with friends, even though I'm people-oriented. I had no sexual energy." A pause. "That's not like me. My incontinence was so bad that I was wearing Depends, but the memory lapses were even more humiliating. I'd sit down with a monthly expense sheet at work and just go blank, have no idea why I'd picked it up or what I was looking for."

It was the hot flashes, however, that ultimately drove her to her doctor. "He gave me a patch. No questions, no discussion. I'd been going to him for 14 years and he still wasn't listening to me. He made his money delivering babies, and he didn't have time for my picky, pesky questions. I sat there on the table and thought, 'I'm going to dump this guy.'" Like Amanda, Peggy found a woman doctor more empathetic, but it still took two years to get the medication right. "Lots of fiddling, lots of experimentation, and meanwhile the symptoms were coming and going."

Peggy's "fuzzy thinking" was clearly affecting her job, and, reasoning that many women on the managerial level at her company were about her age, she decided to start a support group at the office. She got nowhere fast. "Maybe I was naive about the stigma," she says. "These women didn't even want to talk to their husbands about menopause, much less their boss. They were reluctant to band together and accept the label 'menopausal.' I wanted to invite my doctor in and do a seminar, but the other managers were scared the men would hold it against them, that they'd think, 'Oh God, we've got a bunch of menopausal women running this company.'"

Incapable by her very nature of letting a good idea drop so easily, Peggy began leading discussions for other support groups, doing the program she'd designed for her own co-workers at other offices. The reluctance of her friends to come out of the closet still rankles her. "Professional women need to talk to each other," she says. "They're so busy that they're closed off, but we have to have unity to dissolve the stigma at work.

"The joke is that menopausal women already are running this company, and a lot of other companies, and they're doing a fine job of it. But because these smart, competent women won't acknowledge the fact that they're in menopause, the old stereotypes about weepy, hysterical women roll right along."

Rituals of Perimenopause

Our society provides no rite to mark the passage of perimenopause. We don't go into the woods to commune with nature, stand before an altar in a white dress, or throw each other un-baby showers. There are no dances, chants, or greeting cards to publicly announce that we've reached this particular milestone.

But some of the women with whom we spoke devised rituals of their own, personal ways to acknowledge that something in their lives had changed. One woman went to China, a place she always swore she'd visit, a trip she'd canceled after she had become engaged years earlier. Three friends, along with their adult daughters, retraced the grand tour that the older women had taken of Europe after their college graduation 30 years earlier. Now a framed picture of the seven women on the Spanish Steps hangs beside the circa 1964 picture of the older three as young women, standing on the same steps in the same pose, laughing and squinting into the same blazing Italian sun.

Sometimes the rituals were not ones of closure, but sprang from a desire to do something completely new. After menopause, some women felt a sudden zing of energy that prompted them to take up sports or hobbies, sign up for classes, audition for a play at the local theater, or move to a new house. One woman changed the spelling of her first name.

Peggy, the woman we met earlier, threw a slumber party to celebrate her fiftieth birthday. "I definitely planned the party to be symbolic," she says. "It was all about letting go and moving on to the next stage of life. I invited only women to come, even though I'd recently remarried and my new husband had a little problem with that. He wanted to know if he just couldn't stop by when we cut the cake, but I said that this party was to celebrate all the things women do when they're alone together. I was very selective, chose the best friends from all the different aspects of my life without worrying about whether or not everyone knew each other."

A friend who owned a vintage clothing store brought over all of her finery, and after the women played dress-up and each chose a fancy hat, Peggy read aloud the valentines she'd written for her friends over the previous weeks. "I told each friend what was special about her and how important she'd been in my life. After I finished, everyone was crying, and they said, 'It's your birthday. We should have made valentines for you.'

"I'd anticipated that, so I took them into my study where I'd set out all sorts of craft stuff—construction paper, doilies, glitter and ribbons, and glue—and I let them make valentines for me. That was a very important part of the ritual, the single biggest issue I've had to come to grips with lately. I used to try to do everything for everybody else, but in this stage of life I'm going to let other people do nice things for me."

As the evening wore on, the silliness accelerated. The women played relay races, passed LifeSavers on toothpicks, braided each other's hair, told ghost stories, watched movies late into the night, and finally dozed in sleeping bags. The next morning they made pancakes for breakfast and went home. "It was one of the happiest days of my life," says Peggy. "The ritual worked. I keep the valentines in a big box, and I read them when I get down to remind myself how many friends I have, how loved I really am."

12

⚘

Perimenopause: Have It Your Way

Forever is composed of nows.

—Emily Dickinson

We're not trying to suggest that if you follow every piece of advice in this book, life will be perfect or menopause will be easy. The best strategy is to get as much information as you can and approach the experience with an open mind. Women who are determined never to take HRT are rather like the women who enter childbirth vowing that they'll do it "naturally" no matter what. Don't set yourself up for disappointment. Menopause, like childbirth, is different for everyone. You may sail through it, or problems may arise that you couldn't foresee; if so, seeking medical intervention doesn't make you a failure.

But just as you shouldn't reject HRT out of hand, nor should you consider it a panacea. Sedentary, overweight women or those who have been unhappy with their marriages and relationships for years need to address the true roots of their problems and not look to medication to mask the symptoms. It may be tempting to treat estrogen as the "easy answer" to all midlife problems, but no pill can eradicate your need to eat a healthy diet, exercise, and take charge of your own life.

Here are some sample patients and some treatment alternatives they might consider. Although none of these mythic patients is likely to match your exact personal scenario, the point is that you, and your doctor, have options. You should be able to find many ways to handle a problem, and never have to submit to a treatment or regime that makes you uncomfortable.

Patient A

Patient A is a 52-year-old woman who has had no periods for six months, occasional hot flashes, no family history of heart disease, unknown family history concerning osteoporosis and Alzheimer's disease.

The first thing this woman should do is schedule a DEXA. Assuming that her bones are normal, she might:

1. Opt against HRT. Increase exercise, especially weight-resistance training, supplement her diet with 1,500 mg a day of calcium, consider taking soy, reevaluate her diet for fat content, and have her bone density rechecked in two years.

2. If she has a family history of breast cancer, she might follow the plan in number 1, but include raloxifene.

3. Follow the plan in number 1 and add low-dose HRT such as Prempro or the Combipatch (if she can put up with the possibility of breakthrough bleeding) or Estrace 0.5 mg, Premarin 0.3 mg, or Estratab 0.3 mg with cyclic progesterone/progestin.

Patient B

Patient B is 50 years old, has periods every three to six weeks, hot flashes that grow especially strong just before her periods, night sweats, and sleep disturbance. Bone density is unknown, and she does not exercise. Her mother had breast cancer at age 60, but did not take estrogen.

This patient needs a full medical workup, including a DEXA, cholesterol test, and a heart disease risk factor assessment. She should start an exercise program immediately, and then, to relieve her symptoms, she can consider these options:

1. If her DEXA and heart disease tests check out okay, she could take low-dose birth control pills until menopause, and then switch to HRT.

2. If she has any heart disease risk, she might consider cyclic HRT with the progesterone/progestin added the last 12 days of the menstrual cycle. This will regulate her periods and reduce hot flashes.

3. Postmenopausal breast cancer in your mother is not considered a contraindication for HRT, but many women with a history of family breast cancer are understandably fearful. If this is the case for Patient B, she could try soy for her hot flashes and cyclic progestin to control the irregular periods.

Patient C

Patient C is 45 and was diagnosed with breast cancer at age 40. She has ovarian failure induced by chemotherapy, with symptoms including hot flashes and severe vaginal dryness. She has no family history of heart disease or Alzheimer's, and her bone density is normal.

1. Try either soy or Remifemin to reduce the hot flashes. Use an Estring for vaginal dryness. Begin an exercise program, including weight-resistance training, and take calcium supplements. Check regularly for changes in bone density and cholesterol,

and test for colon cancer, which is more common in women who have had breast cancer.

2. Many doctors think HRT does not promote breast cancer in women who have been disease-free for five years. If Patient C's symptoms are making her life miserable, she might opt to take HRT in the lowest possible dosage, along with the lifestyle changes recommended in number 1.

3. She could try raloxifene to prevent bone loss and protect the heart, clonidine for the hot flashes, and an Estring in combination with a lubricant like Astroglide for the vaginal dryness. (Note: It's not clear how soy interacts with SERMs, so it isn't recommended in combination with raloxifene.) Follow the lifestyle changes recommended in number 1.

Patient D

Patient D is 59 years old and has had no symptoms and no periods for eight years; she is active, enjoys normal body weight and a good diet with adequate calcium. However, a DEXA shows osteoporosis in both hip and spine.

1. Take Fosamax 10 mg daily and consult with a physical therapist to begin a program of weight-resistance exercises and ensure proper form. Also take soy supplements with extra calcium.

2. Start HRT using higher doses of estrogen—such as Premarin 1.25 mg daily, Climara or Vivelle 0.1 mg, Estrace 2 mg daily, and so on—to build bone. (Lower dosages of estrogen or drugs such as raloxifene are adequate to maintain bone, but Patient D needs to build bone.) Recheck bone density in one year and, if it isn't increasing, add Fosamax 10 mg per day.

3. Once a DEXA shows that bone density has improved, Fosamax could be decreased or discontinued and the estrogen dose can also be reduced. Continue weight-resistance exercises.

Patient E

Patient E is 39 years old. She suffers PMS with sleep disturbance, irritability, and lethargy. She has had headaches throughout adult life that are especially bad three to five days before her period. Now these PMS-like symptoms are extending up to two weeks before her period and sometimes don't end when her period starts. Periods are unpredictable, ranging from 23 to 28 days apart.

1. Low-dose birth control pills, especially those balanced with more estrogen than progestin, may help regulate the menstrual cycles, as well as reducing the heightened PMS symptoms. Mircette, the birth control pill with the estrogen-only pills on the week of the period would be a good choice.

2. Prozac, or one of the other serotonin-retaining antidepressants, can be taken for the two weeks before the period. You can use birth control pills and Prozac together.

3. An estrogen patch (in a 0.05 mg dosage to start) can be applied for two weeks before the period. This may regulate the periods without necessitating the use of progestin.

4. Use these symptoms as a wake-up call to emphasize exercise, which elevates mood, and eliminate caffeine and alcohol during the worst PMS symptoms.

It's also important to remember that you are likely to be living decades past menopause, and if you want to maintain a comfortable standard of living you should have a personal fiscal plan in place. Your 40s are a good time to consult a financial planner and, much as you did with your doctor, analyze where you are now and what you'll need to do to make sure you stay in good shape during the years to come. It's possible to live a long time through sheer luck. But to live well for a long time you must have a plan.

As we move forward into the new millennium, 4,000 women are entering menopause each day, and as our numbers grow, so does the strength of our voice. We have the right to expect that our complaints be taken seriously, that women's illnesses receive as much funding and research as men's, and that support systems exist to help us through menopause and beyond. We can and should fulfill many of these expectations for ourselves, but some require acknowledgment from the larger community.

The first step in getting what we need is to admit that we need it. As Peggy pointed out in the previous chapter, as long as we are reluctant to claim the word *menopausal,* we're perpetuating the myths. We need to be more vocal about our expectations, especially to our own doctors, and take heart from the fact that our very numbers guarantee we won't be ignored. Although menopause may once have changed women, this generation has the opportunity to change menopause.

Sources

American Cancer Society
19 West 56th St.
New York, NY 10019
(212) 586-8700
www.cancer.org

Among other things, the society offers information on giving up smoking.

American College of Ob Gyn
Office of Public Information
409 12th St. NW
Washington, DC 20024-2188
(202) 638-5577
www.acog.org

Publishes newsletters, pamphlets, and a list of physicians specializing in childbirth and women's diseases.

American Society for Reproductive Medicine
1209 Montgomery Hwy.
Birmingham, AL 35216-2809
(205) 978-5000
www.asrm.org

Call or write for a listing of reproductive endocrinologists as well as information on perimenopausal fertility.

American Lung Association
1740 Broadway
New York, NY 10019
(212) 315-8700
www.lungusa.org

Offers information on giving up smoking.

Association of Applied Biofeedback
10200 West 44th Ave., Suite 304
Wheat Ridge, CO 80033
(303) 422-8436
www.aapb.org

Offers guidance on where to find a biofeedback center or a qualified practitioner as well as general information on the variety of physical disorders that can be improved with this technique.

Good Vibrations
1210 Valencia St.
San Francisco, CA 94110
(800) 289-8423

This legendary San Francisco–based store is a well-known mail-order source of vibrators and other sexual aids.

National Alliance of Breast Cancer Organizations
9 E. 37th St., 10th Floor
New York, NY 10036
(212) 889-0606
www.nabco.org

This is a clearinghouse for the many organizations offering information on breast cancer prevention and treatment, as well as the progress we're making on breast cancer as a national health issue.

National Osteoporosis Foundation
1150 17th St. NW, Suite 500
Washington, DC 20036
(202) 223-2226
www.nof.org

The foundation offers information on calcium, exercise, diagnostic procedures, and the latest research on how to prevent and reverse bone loss.

North American Menopause Society
University Hospitals Department of Ob Gyn
2074 Abington Rd.
Cleveland, OH 44106
(212) 844-3334
www.menopause.org

NAMS can refer you to a local physician with specialized training in menopause and also has a recommended reading list.

Other Web Sites

http://igm.nlm.nih.gov/
www.ama-assn.org/consumer.htm
www.dietarysupplements.info.nih.gov
www.families-first.com
www.mayo.com
www.nih.gov/health

Glossary

Abortion: pregnancy loss, usually before 20 weeks gestation, either spontaneous (naturally occurring) or induced (medically or surgically).

Aerobic exercise: activities requiring oxygen for prolonged periods, improving the body's capacity to handle oxygen.

Amenorrhea: absence of menstrual periods.

Androgens: hormones that produce male characteristics.

Antioxidant: a substance that inhibits oxidation; vitamins A, C, and E are examples.

Artificial insemination: placement of sperm into the female reproductive tract by means other than sexual intercourse.

Basal body temperature (BBT):   temperature taken immediately upon waking before any activity; this temperature rise coincides with a rise in progesterone level following ovulation. Can be used to determine approximate time of ovulation, either to attempt or to avoid pregnancy.

Body Mass Index (BMI):   expresses the relationship between a person's weight and height. It is calculated as weight in kilograms, divided by height in meters squared.

Calcium: mineral essential to building strong bones and teeth.

Duel energy X-ray absorptiometry (DEXA):   a low-dose X-ray technique for measuring bone density.

Endometriosis: disease where tissue from the lining of the uterus grows in areas outside the uterus.

Endometrium: hormonally responsive lining of the uterus cavity; shed every nonpregnant cycle as menstruation.

Estradiol: primary and most potent estrogen produced by the ovaries.

Estrogen: female hormone produced by the ovaries during reproductive years.

Estrone: a weak estrogen derived from estradiol.

Fallopian tube: tube extending from the ovary to the uterus that acts as conduit for sperm to the egg.

Fecundity: the ability to achieve pregnancy (resulting in a live birth) within one menstrual cycle.

Fertility: the ability to conceive and bear a child.

Follicle: saclike structure within the ovary containing an egg.

Follicle-stimulating hormone (FSH):   primary hormone that stimulates the ovary to mature follicles for ovulation; associated with increasing estrogen production throughout the menstrual cycle. An elevated FSH is a sign of menopause.

Formication: tingling sensation on the skin; rare symptom associated with menopause.

HDL cholesterol: smallest and most dense of the substances that transport fats in the blood. Often referred to as "good" cholesterol, because high levels of HDL are protective against cardiovascular disease.

Hormone: chemical messenger produced by a special tissue; it is released into the blood and then travels to distant cells where it exerts its specific effect.

Hormone replacement therapy (HRT): use of estrogen, progesterone, and testosterone to supply the body with hormones that the ovary no longer makes after menopause.

Hysterectomy: surgical removal of the uterus; a "complete" hysterectomy refers to the removal of the tubes and uterus along with the ovaries.

Infertility: one year of unprotected intercourse without conception.

Intracytoplasmic Sperm Injection (ICSI) an extension of IVF where your partner's sperm is placed directly in the egg to accomplish fertilization.

In vitro fertilization (IVF): fertilization of an egg by sperm in a laboratory dish or test tube with placement of the resultant embryo into the woman's uterus.

Isoflavones: phytoestrogens found in soy, garbanzo beans and other legumes.

Kegel exercises: exercise in which one contracts the muscles around the urethra, bladder, and rectum to improve control of urination.

Laparoscopy: surgical procedure using long, thin telescope to view the internal reproductive organs.

LDL cholesterol: low-density lipoprotein carrying cholesterol to blood vessel walls. Often referred to as "bad cholesterol," because high levels of LDL are associated with increased risk of coronary disease.

Libido: sex drive.

Lignans: phytoestrogens that are components of plant cell walls; rich sources include seed oils, particularly flax seed.

Mammogram: X ray of the breast to screen for cancer.

Menarche: occurrence of first menstrual period.

Menopause: cessation of menstruation due to depletion of ovarian follicles (eggs); the end of a woman's ability to reproduce.

Menstrual cycle: a woman's monthly reproductive cycle, with stimulation of ovarian follicular growth and ovulation, corresponding hormone production and resultant thickening of the uterine lining, and shedding of this lining as a menstrual period if pregnancy does not occur.

Oophorectomy: surgical removal of the ovaries.

Osteoporosis: thinning of bone from loss of calcium.

Ovarian failure: inability of the ovary to produce estrogen and progesterone, loss of follicles containing eggs; menopause.

Ovary: organ in the female containing eggs and producing sex hormones.

Ovulation: release of an egg from the ovary.

Perimenopause: transition years leading up to the last menstrual period or menopause.

Phytoestrogens: naturally-occurring plant compounds that may exert effects similar to estrogen; i.e., isoflavones and lignans.

Premenstrual syndrome (PMS):   physical and psychological symptoms associated with the postovulatory phase of the menstrual cycle. Usually followed by a time free of symptoms.

Progesterone: hormone produced by the ovary after ovulation.

Progestin: synthetic hormone with progesterone-like effects; used along with estrogen in HRT.

Progestogen: another term for progestin, a substance acting as progesterone in the body.

Reproductive endocrinology: study of hormonal regulation or reproduction and the menstrual cycle.

Selective Estrogen Receptor Modulators (SERMS): sometimes called "designer estrogens"; they work as estrogen in some tissues in the body and as anti-estrogens in others.

Stress incontinence: involuntary loss of urine with a cough or sneeze.

Tamoxifen: drug that acts as anti-estrogen, countering the effects of estrogen; used in the prevention and treatment of breast cancer.

Testosterone: male hormone produced by the testes in men and, in small amounts, by the ovary in women.

Transdermal: through the skin.

Uterus: female organ in which the fetus develops and is carried throughout a pregnancy. The opening of the uterus in the vagina is the cervix.

Vagina: birth canal, leading from the uterus/cervix to the outside of a woman's body.

Vaginal atrophy: thinning of the vaginal walls due to lack of estrogen.

Weight-bearing exercise: any activity in which the body is forced to support its own weight, such as walking.

Weight-training exercise: physical activity requiring contraction of a muscle and then movement of a joint or extremity against a weight or force (such as a machine, free weights, or a resistance band).

Zygote: an egg that has been fertilized by a sperm.

Index